THE
INTIMACY
FACTOR

THE INTIMACY FACTOR

The Ground Rules
for Overcoming the Obstacles
to Truth, Respect,
and Lasting Love

PIA MELLODY

AND

LAWRENCE S. FREUNDLICH

HarperSanFrancisco
A Division of HarperCollinsPublishers

THE INTIMACY FACTOR: *The Ground Rules for Overcoming the Obstacles to Truth, Respect, and Lasting Love.* Copyright © 2003 by Pia Mellody and Lawrence S. Freundlich. All rights reserved. Printed in the United States of America. No part of this book may be used or reproduced in any manner whatsoever without written permission except in the case of brief quotations embodied in critical articles and reviews. For information address HarperCollins Publishers, Inc., 10 East 53rd Street, New York, NY 10022.

HarperCollins books may be purchased for educational, business, or sales promotional use. For information please write: Special Markets Department, HarperCollins Publishers, Inc., 10 East 53rd Street, New York, NY 10022.

HarperCollins Web site: http://www.harpercollins.com
HarperCollins®, 📖®, and HarperSanFrancisco™ are
trademarks of HarperCollins Publishers, Inc.

FIRST HARPERCOLLINS PAPERBACK EDITION
PUBLISHED IN 2004.
Designed by Joseph Rutt
Library of Congress Cataloging-in-Publication Data available upon request.
ISBN 0–06–009580–6 (paperback)
07 08 ❖ RRD(H) 10 9 8 7 6

To Pat Mellody, who has encouraged my work and challenged my thinking over the more than twenty years we have worked together. He has always believed that I could accomplish great things.

CONTENTS

ACKNOWLEDGMENTS

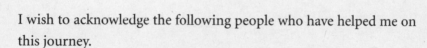

I wish to acknowledge the following people who have helped me on this journey.

The many people who have been willing to do the healing work that is necessary in the recovery process.

Larry Freundlich, who so expertly has given words to my thoughts in the production of this book.

Bob and Maurine Fulton, who demonstrate in their lives and in their therapy that intimacy can be both possible and comfortable.

Terry Real and Belinda Berman, with whom I have worked for many years and who have helped me to develop.

Mona Sides Smith and Monique Laughlin, two fine therapists who have worked with me to prove the effectiveness of my ideas.

INTRODUCTION

My essential reason for writing *The Intimacy Factor* is to acknowledge the role of spirituality in intimate relationships. By spirituality I mean the acknowledgment of and trust in a power greater than the self. Under the proper conditions, spirituality restores to us to a sense of the inalienable inherent worth with which we were born and with which we lost contact through trauma and adaptation.

Once recovering persons acknowledge the truth of who they are and feel love for themselves in the face of that truth, they are prepared to recognize it in others. They now have a personal spiritual template that guides their vision to perceive other spiritual realities in the world, the most important of which is other people, whom they now recognize as having, like themselves, inherent worth. It changes the way they treat people and the way they are treated in return. This ultimately is what makes intimate relationships possible, and it makes them work.

The recognition of this truth finally makes intimacy possible; we are reattached to the beneficent processes of life that were ours at birth. That is when the amazing discovery of the spiritual path is felt. That is when the presence of a Higher Power becomes a personal reality. For me, this relationship with a Higher Power is the most important fact of my life.

My first awareness of a spiritual connection came long before I had begun to study the mechanisms of childhood abuse and the process of healing from it. God's presence in my life came to me through revelation, and I consider it a miracle, because it came unbidden. Indeed, when I had this experience of God, I was an emotional wreck and unable to care for myself, much less have a relationship worthy of the name.

Why or how revelation occurs is beyond human understanding. It is not the subject of this book—it could not be. But in saving my life, the Higher Power set me on a path of self-analysis and study of other sufferers that taught me how to guide people to the healing moment. Finally, I learned how to create for others the conditions under which self-understanding, true relationships, intimacy, and spirituality are possible. Truth about self and respect for the truth of others are the portals through which true intimacy and spirituality enter. No intimate relationship is possible without them, and spirituality is a gift of relationship.

At the center of this discovery is the concept of boundaries that create the experience of truth and respect. The system of boundaries that I teach enables each of us to maintain our inherent worth in the face of all outside pressures, rarely allowing the opinions or emotions of others to erode our belief in our inherent worth. Secure in our own self-worth, we do not feel so threatened, diminished, or shamed by others. We do not have to make defensive or offensive adaptations to maintain our dignity. It is in such a state that true relationships are possible. For most of us, achieving this state is one of the most delicate and often painful achievements of adulthood. Most of us find our greatest pain and disappointment in relationships that we cannot make work.

When we are in a relationship, we are called on to give body, thoughts, and emotions to our partners and to accept body, thoughts, and emotions from them. Learning how to do this is a pre-requisite for intimacy and the spirituality to which it gives birth. To do it badly causes misery. To do it well honors the best part of our humanity and puts us in psychological balance, which results in a sense of connectedness with life's goodness.

When we are in the experience of the truth of self, we know that the self has inherent worth. As we are in relationship—whether by listening or touching or feeling emotions—we must be willing to face the truth of the other person and be able to love, or at minimum respect, the other's own inherent worth, apart from the way he or she behaves. That is spiritual. It starts with our partners, children, friends, lovers, and adversaries and reaches outwards toward God. Since relating to our fellow humans goes on almost every moment of our lives, the practice of healthy relationships not only puts us on a spiritual path; it keeps us there.

They say that the spiritual path is straight and narrow, but I used to wonder about that. I used to think that the spiritual path was about being good. It was hard to be good because there were only a few ways of being good. I have since learned the opposite. The spiritual path is straight and narrow because all it takes is moving into a lie to make you absolutely step off of it. I made this discovery when I was trying to teach people to be intimate with one another in their relationships. It was in that effort that I formulated my theory of boundaries.

By recovering from the psychological damage that keeps us from intimacy, we learn to experience renewed self-esteem, personal power, and faith, which give us the ability to have intimate relation-ships in the first place. This book will identify those ghosts of the past and, by throwing the light of truth upon them, clear the path toward intimacy in relationships. It will teach the psychological tech-niques by which intimacy is maintained on behalf of the self, the ones we love, and the ones we want to love us. The most important lesson of this book is teaching people how to love and be loved.

Achieving intimacy is like tuning in a radio station. At first there is a lot of buzzing and indistinguishable noise; then you find the signal and can hear clearly. If you continue turning the dial, however, you lose the signal. Through the years I found two things that clearly tune in the radio station: one is truth and the other one is love. When we tell ourselves the truth instead of lies, we are automatically tuning in Higher Power energy. In choosing truth, we choose to be loving to self and others; then the radio station is absolutely, perfectly clear.

Love is a continuum that ranges all the way from respect to very warm regard, the latter of which most people call "love." For many years I mistakenly thought that if I loved someone, all I needed to do was to continually have a deep sense of warmth for him. Although that deep sense of warmth is basic, there are also other degrees of love that have to do with the condition of the relationship. As we experience the truth of another person, that person may be difficult—human. We might naturally feel fear, pain, and shame—not exactly pleasant. I had the idea that if I felt these unpleasant emotions, I was not loving the other person. And early on actually I wasn't, but as I recovered I began to feel something healthy in its place. I learned to recognize another ingredient, and that was respect. If I could consciously hold on to my awareness of the other's inherent worth, while that person was being difficult and I was feeling angry, he would feel respect coming from me, and I would feel respect coming back from him.

The emotions we experience in relationship with humans operate also when we seek intimacy with God. When you are in relationship with God, you are being intimate with God, which is like being intimate with anyone else. You share the self, the body, the mind;

you share your emotions; you let your behavior be seen; you reveal yourself. And you stand and receive the self of another. You give and receive with humans in your healthy relationships with them and you do the same with God in prayer and meditation, and in some instances in revelation.

When I am in relationship with God, I get what I need, even if I don't know what I need. I receive a variety of things, foremost among them the sense of being loved unconditionally. Another is direction, guidance, what to do, what not to do, what is needed. The third thing is a sense of solace and relief from the burdens of being a human on this planet. I get a sense of balance; I sense that all is well. The fourth thing I can receive is grace, which I call automatic healing. Often I experience something about myself that is less than perfect, that I would like to overcome, such as anger, fear, or shame. Grace is the experience of God that keeps me from being compelled to act out that anger, fear, or shame. It doesn't even occur to me to do so. I have peace of mind.

The work of humans and the work of God seemingly go hand in hand. When through the concrete psychological process of discovery that I describe in this book, truth about the self is set free to nourish our relationships, we find that intimate relationality itself is the path of the spirit and entitles us to God's several gifts, chief among which is love.

One of the most fundamental maxims of twelve-step recovery is that it is a "We Program." That means that dysfunctional people seeking peace and fulfillment find the solutions together. They learn from one another. Being able to learn from and to teach another human being requires having a relationship with him or her. Yet all healthy relationships require of each partner knowledge of the true self. The first step in my treatment is the discovery of the truth: the truth about the core issues that drive the patient's dysfunction.

Without truth there can be no intimacy, because without truth you wind up sharing lies or delusions. Without intimacy there can be no relationship. When two partners share their true selves, protecting self and other by the correct practice of boundaries, the miracle of spirituality is present. It is the journey from truth to intimacy to relationship to spirituality that this book will describe.

It has taken me twenty-five years to formulate what I have learned and experienced about dysfunction and recovery. The events of my life that brought me to a spiritual bottom were rooted in my childhood, but at the stage of my life when I was helplessly tortured by them, I had no rational way to start my way on the road to recovery. I acknowledge that I was put on the spiritual path by an epiphany, and understanding came later. However, when the spiritual path became open to me, it led me to formulate a psychology that can be taught and learned even by those in the greatest pain. I had to wait for an inexplicable spiritual event in my life, but you do not. I want you to get there much faster than I did—along a much more predictable path.

THE
INTIMACY
FACTOR

1

A SPIRITUAL
HOMECOMING

But as I rav'd and grew more fierce and wilde
At every word,
Me thought I heard one calling, Childe:
And I reply'd, My Lord.
          —George Herbert, "The Collar"

Those of us in twelve-step recovery learn that the most pernicious effect of our addictions and the psychic disorders that come along with them is spiritual isolation. We feel that we have become "terminally unique." Everywhere we turn we find ourselves at the center of a hostile universe against which we must defend ourselves by dishonesty or hostility or withdrawal. We are defiant or abashed, and always we feel shame. This egocentricity makes us feel that "everyone is looking at us" and that we have to do something about it or suffer. We call this "self-centered fear." One of the witticisms of AA describes a person in this state as being "an arrogant doormat" or as "that piece of garbage around which the entire universe revolves."

Rejoining the human race with a proper understanding of our interdependence is the task we work on from the time we attend our first AA meeting. And no better way has been found for us to begin that task of reuniting with our fellow humans than in listening to their stories and in telling our own. I would like to share my story with you.

When I was an infant, my father was away at war, and my mother was overwhelmed by being a single parent. She would have breakdowns, during which she would sleep the morning away and leave my sister to play by herself and me to anguish in my crib, unfed and uncared-for, until she got up. Sometime between my third and fourth years I was molested by a gang of boys. These abuses were stamped like fossilized footprints in my soul. I was traumatized at an age so young that I had no language skills to shield me from the immediate, visceral pain. That pain and the memory of my early childhood wounds remained beyond my recall for many years.

When I was approximately seven years old, I realized that my mother was preoccupied with fighting with my father. When I complained to her about him, however, she denied that there was anything wrong with him. My reality was unreliable, she implied—illusory. As for my father, he could not stand the sound and sight of me, and he told me so, without shame. When he wasn't demeaning me, he ignored me. I felt worthless, hopeless, and frightened. I had trouble sleeping, and I had nightmares.

No longer the passive, blank slate that I was as a three- and four-year-old, I thought up tactics to help me survive in this abusive family system. I now had language and concepts to help me cope. If reality was unacceptably painful for me, I would make up my own.

What I did to survive was to go silent; I "disappeared." I spent time away from the house and told my parents nothing about what I was doing. I didn't want to be noticed. Worse than being a lost child, I became the irrelevant child. My parents knew where I was—unfortunately for me, I had no place in their plans.

When I was about thirteen, my mother began to relate details about how awful, how sadistic, my father was to her and threatened divorce. The more she began to unburden herself, the more I began to feel afraid for myself and for her. I was overwhelmed by a feeling of responsibility for her and felt as if I had to save her. The more she made me the repository of her complaints, the more she seemed like a helpless child, the victim of my father; and the more childlike she seemed, the more "adult" and "better than" I became. I also felt angry and confused as I remembered my mother's earlier denial of my complaints about my father—the very same man she was now telling me was so sadistic.

Also, at this time, I was approaching adolescence and having a hard time dealing with teenage boys. I felt frightened and repulsed, not knowing that their sexuality was stirring up the emotional intimations of my childhood molestation. All these wounds and the adaptations I made to tolerate them took up residence within me— unexamined, untreated, free to twist and distort my soul.

As an adult, when I first began to study the problem of childhood abuse and treatment, I found that a man or woman who was important to me could remind me of either my mother or my father and send me spinning back to those emotions and wounds I had received through infancy, childhood, and adolescence. Real relationships—I had none. The specific ages at which I had experienced abuse had created ego states, each with its own characteristics. The three-year-old was frightened and helpless; the seven-year-old was extremely depressed, felt shame-filled, worthless, and alone; and the thirteen-year-old was filled with fear, confusion, and anger.

When these wounds were stimulated, each one had a different voice in my head. Each troubled voice came from a part of me that had received a significant wounding. It would take many years of suffering and bewilderment before I could even remember or focus on and accept my trauma history.

But that painful day did come. One day my older sister recounted for me the details of the abuse I had known as a baby. It was the first time ever that I had experienced the reality of that early wounding. The shock to my psyche was tremendous. Before my sister's eyes, I was helplessly plunged back into a very early, prelanguage, wounded-child state. My mind and emotions swirled out of control. I was completely overwhelmed with a sense of spinning apart. I lay down and curled up into a ball in order to stop the spinning.

As a child I had worked desperately to be good so that I could avoid feeling so worthless. For me to be good was the only solace I had for the fear and the pain. As an abused child, I was treated by my family as if I were irrelevant, and that was who in my mind and heart I had become—a misfit. Only by retreating into my hermetic world of self-definition could I force myself to believe that I was worth being loved and cared for.

Unfortunately, my notion of being good forced me never to admit that anything was wrong. It made it seem to my parents that I had no problems, so my adaptation made them even less aware of me. But even if they had listened to me, my parents were too damaged to have helped.

By trying to be perfect, I was denying my perfectly imperfect humanity. I believed that if others saw who I "really" was, they would find me pitiful. My self-esteem had become so compromised that hiding out was the only way I could avoid shame attacks. Because trying to be perfect had not made me feel better, I had tried to find some solace in various churches. But my attempts to find a relationship with God had been a failure and by the time I was fourteen, my attempts to get relief through religion were exhausted. I blamed my own deficiencies for my failure to find a God who could solace me, deepening my own sense of worthlessness.

Afflicted as I was with damaged self-esteem, I tried to lead my life as best I could while toting around my dysfunctions like an invisible knapsack. Eventually, like many people who cannot find solutions to their personal problems within their own souls and who search for a "rescuer," I got married, and, predictably, I discovered that no one, not even a husband, could do for me what I could not do for myself. Apart from whatever difficulties the marriage held for me, I became more and more depressed. I wasn't suicidal, but I was miserable. I began to believe that I was beyond help—crazy.

I got so desperate in that misery that I turned to my mother-in-law. She had always described herself as a fundamentalist Christian, and I found her to be controlling, critical, and superior to me. Nonetheless, I asked her if she could help me with my depression. I allowed myself to fall into the orbit of her intense religious energies, and with her support I turned my will and my life over to the care of God. However, my depression, although somewhat lightened, still remained with me.

During the time that I had this religious experience, I did not believe in God, and I do not think that I came to believe in God. What did happen was that I, a disbeliever, developed some experience of faith that was enough for me to be able to step onto the spiritual path. Apparently, there is a space between disbelieving and truly believing when we understand the limitations of our humanity and receive the gift of spirituality.

Despite these spiritual intimations, my life worsened until it got to the point that I wanted to end it. It was then that I experienced an epiphany. I was suddenly surrounded by what felt to me like the presence of God. I felt completely embraced and could hear this energy communicating to me—not like normal conversation—but like pure communication. What the energy communicated to me was that I was immobilized by fear and had become unable to embrace life. That was why I felt suicidal.

This energy told me that if I faced my fears and did what was in front of me—what I didn't want to do—I would get the backup, the support, and the very means of working my way out—of changing what was going on in my life. At the same time that I knew I had to embrace my fear, I was experiencing an extraordinary sense of unconditional love coming from this Power greater than myself. As I experienced that love, I began, for the first time in my life, to feel self-love. Because this experience was so profoundly moving, I came to believe that I could be in a relationship with God and that God loved me and would back me up. So I set out to do what needed to be done, and as I did that, I became part of the solution rather than part of the problem.

I eventually became a nurse working at a drug and rehabilitation facility in Wickenburg, Arizona. In addition to my nursing duties, I started listening to the lectures on addiction. The complaints I heard the alcoholic patients sharing with one another sounded as if the patients were privy to my own emotional pain, and I came to understand that I was an alcoholic.

As my knowledge and intuition about the underlying causes of alcoholism grew, I myself was still in the grips of psychological dysfunctions that had had their origins in my childhood. Despite my growing awareness of the problems of the patients, I remained helpless to care for myself.

I remember the first moment I acknowledged that to myself. I was listening to a friend of mine lecture on what alcoholism was, and I remember saying to her that I thought I was an alcoholic, that I had the symptoms she was talking about. And I remember her saying, "Well, welcome." It was as if she knew all along and had been waiting for me to discover it by myself. When she said that to me, I felt as if I had come home. I felt joy-pain, or tears of joy. It was as if my whole psyche or soul had relaxed, and I felt at home—as if in a community with people like me.

I started becoming involved in the treatment of alcoholics, and I was asked to help in developing ways of treating chemical dependencies and other psychological problems. When I was asked to do this, I felt quite inadequate. I also felt angry because I was a nurse and I thought that the counselors, therapists, and doctors should be addressing these issues, not me. As my resistance grew, I had a powerful epiphany similar to the one I had had when I was suicidal.

What was communicated to me was that I needed to do what was being asked of me and that I would get the help I needed. What started happening was that when I was meditating, I would receive information about how to treat the problems of patients.

The program director had heard reports from staff and patients of my sudden impatience and losses of temper. Any kind of criticism could trigger my sense of worthlessness and drive me to defend myself by lashing out. On several occasions, I had complained directly to him in an inappropriately overwrought manner; and he not only described in detail the extent of my bizarre attitudes but became increasingly concerned that I do something about them. He was willing to give me time. He had a faith in me that I didn't yet have in myself.

Yet I could see clearly in the patients what I was having difficulty facing in myself. That is when I began to get glimmers and insights into a system of issues that lay at the heart of the dysfunctional psyche, a system that had been put in place in the childhoods of the patients as well as in my own.

At the core of this system, I identified issues of *self-esteem, boundaries, reality, self-care,* and *moderation.* I noticed that in dealing with each one of these core issues, the dysfunctional adult tended to act in the extreme. If we looked at the self-esteem issue, for example, I saw that the patients wobbled back and forth between thinking that they were either worthless or "better than," between feeling too vulnerable and feeling invulnerable. They would feel bad about themselves to the point of self-detestation or, through the delusion of perfectionism, bestow upon themselves a sense of irreproachable goodness. Some patients would feel too dependent, wanting others to take care of them. But other patients seemed to be antidependent or needless and wantless—refusing to accept help or to admit that they had any needs at all. Some patients were walled in and couldn't express their truth; others were at the other extreme and spewed thoughts and emotions. Some patients acted childishly and immaturely while others seemed overly mature, rigid, and controlling.

Knowing that these extremes were present in me, I began to remember what it was like to receive treatment from medical people who were ignorant of the causes of these extremes, and—what was so aggravating for me to recognize—ignorant of their own entrapment within them.

Although the patients' dysfunction was usually out in the open and easily recognizable, a like set of dysfunctions was present among the health-care professionals but always went undetected. The dysfunctions of the health-care professionals were usually the exact opposite of the dysfunctions of the patients. If the patient was one-down (low self-esteem), the health-care professional was one-up (high self-esteem). If the patient was boundaryless, the professional was walled in (strong or invulnerable). If the patient was filled with a sense of imperfection, the professional was perfect, needless and wantless, and in control of everything (rigid). In the general culture, these dysfunctional characteristics of the health-care professional passed as mental health—the mark of a good doctor.

"Neurotic patients" lived in the extremes of "less than": vulnerable, self-loathing, inexpressive of personal reality, overdependent, needy, immature. These people were often called "crazy." But the caregivers who were trying to help these people had the same issues, only at the "better than" end of the extreme. Their one-up issue was a self-esteem issue; their invulnerability was a boundary problem; their perfectionism was a reality issue; their antidependence was a self-care issue; their controlling rigidity was a moderation issue. Their having walls for boundaries was a boundary problem because it prevented intimacy.

With the insight that the medical professionals were caught up in the same dysfunctions as their patients, my resistance to doing this healing and learning work was lifted. I recognized that I hadn't wanted to be a "healer" because healers themselves were causing pain through their own dysfunction and were blinded to it by their sense of superiority. With knowledge that the core issues yielded self-knowledge, it would be possible to be a therapist and a true healer.

What I had come to see was that without a respectful relationship between the patient and the healer there could be no change or growth for the patient. For patient and healer to exchange the kind of candor and truth necessary to effect change in the patient, the healer could not relate from the one-up position to the patient in the one-down position. From inferiority or superiority neither patient nor healer is in his or her authentic self but is caught in the voices and the states of mind of childhood trauma.

That insight helped me discover what is required to be in true relationship. Only healthy selves have the capacity to have true relationships. "Physician, heal thyself" suddenly had vital meaning for me.

Patients were beginning to line up outside my office. They had found someone who understood them, but, perhaps more important, someone who was just like them. Every time we communicated as equals, I was getting help for myself.

I felt great energy, excitement, and passion about what I was doing. It was similar to that feeling of having come home at last that

I had the day I acknowledged that I was an alcoholic. This passion unlocked a part of my meditative mind that enabled me to spend a lot of time thinking about just what these problems were. It may seem comic, but my mind was never more open than when I was vacuuming. When I vacuumed, my mind would be flooded with all kinds of ideas of what the disease was and how to treat it. I found myself writing all this down as it occurred to me. Later I would go back and talk to the patients about my thoughts and feelings, and they would have an amazed reaction to it, telling me that what I was saying was so helpful—that the exact same things were going on with them.

I did not want to be a hypocrite—telling people to live one way, but not doing it myself. I started making myself do all the things that were occurring to me, and I became healthier and felt a lot better. And every time I spoke about the things that were occurring to me, I got bigger reactions to it. Finally the program director complained that there were too many patients trying to get in to see me, and he asked me to take a formal position in the counseling program.

At times I would run into my old resistance and hear, "I told you to do what was in front of you and to face your fears." So then I made myself do the things that I never thought I could or should do in the first place. And it just kind of mushroomed into a huge project that seemed to have helped a lot of people.

What I was led to do was to acknowledge the skews of the psyche in which our inner voices conspire to rob us of our inner worth, and then I started to work on healing those. And in healing those, I became more and more and more aware of the spiritual path. I got help to face the things that I was asked to do but thought I couldn't. And I did them anyway. I always got the help I needed, and I still do. It is amazing.

2

FALSE EMPOWERMENT AND DISEMPOWERMENT

Learning to Be "Better Than," Learning to Be "Less Than"

The ceremony of innocence is drowned;
The best lack all conviction, while the worst
Are full of passionate intensity.
>   —William Butler Yeats,
>   "The Second Coming"

Abusive parenting creates a painful sense of shame, inadequacy, or superiority in children, which, if left unacknowledged and untreated, results in the prolongation of these wounds into adulthood. When events in the life of adults who still carry the wounds of childhood trauma stir up unconscious memories of their original wounding, they reexperience the shame or grandiosity of childhood and respond immaturely and dysfunctionally.

These problems of relationship with their origins in childhood are hidden from view by layer upon layer of dysfunctional adult adaptation, the layers now having usurped the true or authentic self.

In such a state, healthy intimacy is impossible. Healthy intimacy requires the trusting offer of our true self to another and our trusting acceptance of the other's true self in return.

For example, when a colleague of Kim's at work reminded her that her part of the work assignment was due very shortly, she felt shame and masked it with anger. She struck out at him, telling him that she needed no reminder and that if he tended to his own business, things would go a lot more smoothly. She comforted her ego by telling herself, "Nobody screws around with me." Kim's colleague had struck a raw nerve in her. Long ago her parents had taught her that she was unsatisfactory. When her colleague stirred up this old feeling, she struck back at him, coming at him from the place of her old wound.

Traumatized children originally adapted to familial abuse in order to survive within the abusive family system. They believed that only by adapting to their parents' expectations of them would they remain protected. Maintaining the status quo, even if it was a sick status quo, was for these children better than being abandoned or losing their identity within the family. They protected themselves from the primal fear of abandonment even as they lost contact with their true selves. The abusive family they worked so painfully to stabilize by fitting in provoked them to abandon their authenticity. From the point of view of the children, these adaptations were a matter of life and death. Their utility was sanctioned by the most powerful animal instinct: survival.

From the viewpoint of traumatized children, the phrase "matters of life and death" is not a metaphor—it is the urgent reality of their instinct to live. It is irresistible as an instinct, and, short of grace, there is nothing so powerful. The children instinctively feel that they depend on the care of their parents for life. In that life-and-death situation, they must learn to find their place in the life-giving system, even if the hindsight of adulthood shows their adaptation to have been spiritually crippling.

The pain and inadequacy signaled to adults from the ghostly wounds of the past leave them as unprotected and uncomfortable as they were at the time they were first wounded as children. Uncomfortable in their skins, unhappy with their lives, frightened, angry, and resentful of their coworkers, lovers, and families, these people seek relief from suffering and hope for a better life.

One of my patients, Max, a successful director of documentary films, was fluent in English, French, and German and had a Ph.D. in political science from a prestigious European university. He told me something about his father, who was a brilliant and successful man. He said that when he was about seven years old, he asked his grandmother if he could play a certain game while his parents were away for the evening. His grandmother told him that he would have to get permission from his father. When he asked his father for permission, his father said definitely not. My patient then went back to his grandmother and lied to her that his father had given him permission. When his father discovered that his son had lied to the grandmother and disobeyed his orders, he screamed at the child and walked over to the telephone. He picked up the receiver, only pretending to have dialed out. The father made believe he had a reform school on the line. He told the imaginary head of the reform school that he had a very bad boy on his hands and that he and his wife didn't want him anymore. They were packing his bags and would bring him over in the morning. They didn't want to hear anything more about him until he had learned how to behave.

Today Max complains of having little confidence in business negotiations, of being too concerned about the good opinion of his adversary, of feeling that he would lose if he stood up for his rights. His anxiety shows itself by his either becoming tediously legalistic and stilted or by asking for less than is appropriate.

Another patient, Maria, a woman in her middle thirties from a family of millionaire bankers and artists, reports that she has a dead marriage. Her husband never acknowledges his own real emotions. His relationship with her seems cold and perfunctory. He does not understand what she is talking about when she tells him that he is emotionally unavailable. Cut off from emotional sharing with him, she has become his "housekeeper" and the "nanny" to their children. She is depressed, frustrated, and angry. She hates herself for her futility. She knows she has to get a divorce, but she does not know if that would be abandoning her responsibility to the marriage. Perhaps it is all her fault. If she only knew what he wanted, perhaps she could provide it, and then everything would be all right. She has a tendency to ramble on and on, blaming first herself and then others, trying out one insight and then denying it in the next breath. At the end of most of her sentences, her voice loses strength and evaporates into unintelligibility. It seems she doesn't even believe herself.

She tells me that her father, born in Latin America, believed in the subservience of women. As an artist, he had a destiny to fulfill, and his wife and children were there to serve him, to let him do his thing. At the dinner table, he pontificated and was unaware of the needs of my patient or her three younger sisters. Maria's mother was utterly dominated by her husband. She used the family's considerable wealth and privilege to cater to his every need. And his most dramatic need was to be left alone. Not only did he ignore the children except when he was pontificating; he ignored his wife. Maria's mother concentrated all her emotions on my patient. She was over-the-top vivacious, spreading emotion left and right like a fertilizer spreader. Disguised beneath her lavish outpouring of affection, she turned to her daughter to replace her husband's love. She has made Maria a combination of servant and substitute spouse.

Maria became responsible for arranging the family's social schedule; for listening to her mother's complaints; for taking care of her sisters in order to relieve the burden on the mother; and, most painfully, for being the mediator between her needy mother and her dismissive father. She had no life of her own. Her only worth was the worth she got from serving her mother. She was important and lovable only when she sacrificed herself. Enmeshed with her mother, whose life depended on her daughter's devotion, she was programmed to deny her own needs. She associates love with her own needlessness.

After she married, Maria remained in excessive contact with her mother. She was constantly on the phone with her. When her mother bought a large townhouse, Maria and her husband moved into the apartment above the mother, who is always on hand to baby-sit, run errands, and demand services from her daughter in return. It is likely that the emotional distance Maria detects in her husband is similar to the estrangement he feels from her due to her primary attachment to her mother. This enmeshment with her mother makes intimacy between husband and wife impossible. Finding it easier to lay the blame on her husband than on her attachment to her mother, Maria thinks that getting a divorce will solve her problem, freeing her to find a proper soul mate.

Kenneth, a thirty-eight-year-old, successful ("I have the biggest house in town") architect, had repressed the memory of being regularly sexually abused by an older female cousin, abuse that had gone on until he was twelve. In Kenneth's family of origin, the father had died in a car crash, which left the family financially unstable. To him his mother seemed always about to collapse. From the time he was five years old, he took on as many household chores as he could in order to keep his mother going. He was terrified of losing her, his only support in life. He became totally enmeshed in her life, living to keep her alive.

The one happy memory Kenneth had of childhood was of an older cousin who came to visit three times a year. She gave the family money and food and took them on vacations. As he went on about his cousin, he started sobbing. He could barely catch his breath. He was beginning to remember that his cousin sexually abused him and that he thought his mother knew what was going on and had done nothing to stop the abuse. He was now complaining that he felt smothered and panicked whenever he got into an intimate situation with a woman. He is in love now, but is subject to dissociating when he and his girlfriend are feeling sexual. He thinks he will be alone forever.

These vignettes evoke several dysfunctions the origins of which lie in abusive parenting: worthlessness, fear of abandonment, damaged self-esteem, needlessness and wantlessness, the grandiosity of "better than," the remorse of "less than," and the equation of love with suffocation. They are a part of the catalog of the spiritual malaise of our times and, as a result, are also a catalog of prime factors in our inability to achieve and maintain true intimacy.

There are those who fear to assert themselves. Others suffer from being alienated from their children. Some feel the "deadness" in relationships they had hoped would be vital and intimate. They feel incapable of giving or receiving love. There are those whose emotions have gone explosive and who experience out-of-control sexuality, anger, or the tyrannical need to control. Many fear making commitments; they complain of self-loathing or underachievement.

The dysfunctional adult in relationship with another dysfunctional adult trades defense and attack, the firepower for each side being provided by the unacknowledged remnants of childhood abuse. The damaged self, hypnotically reacting to the promptings of the past, becomes cut off from the present, like a prisoner asking for love and support through soundproof glass.

Many of us have been sufficiently compromised by our trauma histories that we cannot function properly under stress. Even when we find temporary private ways to cope with our anxiety (exercise, television, food, travel), we find ourselves breathing the toxic air of a general culture that constantly induces stress—perhaps most destructively by damaging our ability to be functionally mature parents.

In the first rank of modern-day cultural stress inducers is the amount of information available to us and the speed at which it floods over us. This corrodes the self-confidence and ethical convictions on which parental authority is based. Daytime soap operas offer a daily fare of adultery, addiction, rage, and jealousy. Talk-show hosts serve up the private sexual lives of their guests ranging from teenage lesbianism to trailer-park violence to adultery and fetishism. Music videos flaunt sex and hatred of authority and glorify teenage rebellion and rage. Cartoon shows in prime time substitute absurd and wild caricatures of human beings who flaunt the limits of social and family decorum while blurring the line between reality and fantasy. Sports events include no-holds-barred free-for-alls implying maiming and imminent death. Extreme sports glorify preteens driving motorcycles over backbreaking moguls, preparing them and their eager viewers to take the same carelessness onto the superhighway of life. The commercials that support this assault deliver the message that if you buy this or buy that you will be all right: Just keep watching. Just keep buying.

Many of us have become unable to teach our children the right lessons of love and trust because we parents, like our children, were raised in the same culture and were equally corrupted by it. We are just like them. We never grew up. Adults depend on the network news for information about the public sector. And with one exception the news that is most noteworthy is news of international violence, theft, and betrayal of the public trust. The exception is what dress an actress is wearing to the Oscars. If you miss the news one night, there is no need to worry. Tune in tomorrow. It will be the same.

The extended family, which once included grandparents, has largely disappeared, along with the backup they provided for parenting. High divorce rates and single-parent homes have further thinned the ranks of those who previously were counted on to provide education and role models.

The most influential messages of the communications media come through advertising, the covert message of which is that we are inadequate the way we are and need to acquire the products or services being hawked by the advertiser in order fix our deficiency. When we acquire the stuff that is supposed to make us better, we find that it hasn't done the trick, and the stress of inadequacy is increased, making parents uneasy in roles of authority. It is macabre to see both parent and child dressed in the same brand-name sports outfit, watching the same television shows, and listening to the same top-of-the-chart music. Both creatures of the same marketing influences, they wear their matching baseball caps turned backward like their values.

In Wickenburg, Arizona, where I live, you never see people sitting on their porches with their friends. It seems everyone is inside isolating themselves in front of the television set. Basketball teammates, traveling on the school bus to play a local rival, sit in their seats either plugged into a CD music player or watching (the more affluent of them) some violent Hollywood thriller on their DVD player. For all intents and purposes, they might as well be traveling alone. In short, what is missing from my neighborhood, and thousands of others just like it, is a sense of community in which neighbors in daily communication with one another become mutual caregivers and emotional backups for one another.

There is a fascinating history to the word "gossip," which tells us how isolated we have become in our communities. In medieval Ireland, because the men spent the days in the fields and because so many women died in childbirth or of early disease, there were few adults to watch over the children. It became the honored custom for anyone in the community who saw or spoke to a child in the course of the day's work to pass on that information immediately to anyone else in the community. That constant concern with the children was called "gossiping" the children, and it was meant to keep them under the concerned surveillance of the adult community. Now when we ask our children where they are going and the answer comes back "To the mall" or just "Out," that is often where parental control stops. And, of course, "gossip" has become a pejorative word, implying unwarranted interest in another's affairs: it is better not to know what your neighbor is doing.

Under the spur of investigative reporting made available to everyone through the Internet, television, radio, and the newspapers, many of the institutions that used to be the repositories of our pride and ethical certainties have become corroded. Scandal is what makes news.

Under stress it doesn't take too much for people to figure out that obsessive-compulsive use of drugs and alcohol and activities like sex can medicate them. And I include in this list compulsive shopping, risk taking, work addiction, and overeating. These activities momentarily decrease stress before creating tremendous problems that actually increase stress.

Those of us in the addiction-treatment field know that people use their addictive processes as their god, which reduces their stress and provides a short-term solution to their inadequacy. When they discover that the god of their addiction has failed them, rather than giving up their false god, they just switch addictions, which creates chaos and stress all over again.

Stress that destroys our ability to have true relationships and to be mature parents is harder to identify than the dramatic and often bizarre behavior of the substance abuser. However, in the stressful world in which many of us today struggle to raise our children, we tragically although inadvertently traumatize and burden them with pain that may last their entire lives.

To stressed parents the job of parenting can from moment to moment become overwhelming, and those parents, unaware of how inappropriately they are parenting, are often bewildered, saddened, enraged, or depressed by the results. The parents overreact to children and do one of two things that sets up the whole problem: they *falsely empower* or *disempower.*

All trauma results from either disempowering abuse or falsely empowering abuse, which because of its falseness disempowers as well. The abusive parent either shames the child into silence as a way of diminishing his or her own external stress, thereby disempowering the child, or assigns the child roles in which the child performs assignments for which the parent should be responsible, thereby falsely empowering the child. An example of the latter would be a stressed-out mother who, because her relation to her abusive husband is unbearable, turns to her young son, depending on him for love and implying that without his support she will have no one.

Under *false empowerment* children are asked to take care of parents. Parents make the children think that assigning them this role has given them power and importance. In fact, these parents are robbing the children of their childhood. Assigned roles include Hero, Heroine, Mediator, Counselor, Daddy's Little Girl, Mommy's Little Man, and the Mascot, who is used to bringing stress-reducing humor into the family. Burdening children with the job of caring for parents traumatizes the children by silencing their true, or authentic, selves. They wind up with a false sense of value. Their false empowerment makes them "better than" or one-up over the parents they are caring for.

Falsely empowered children have become adapted to playing a role they can never perform without damaging their childhood spontaneity, the authenticity of their youth. These children lose contact with their own humanity but are unaware of the deprivation, and although the children know that something is not quite right, the praise they get for being so good and for making their parents so proud keeps them content in their delusion of power. Parents and children have both lost contact with the truth of what is going on. They are living a lie.

Falsely empowered children's source of value comes from outside. These children never learn the concept of inherent worth. Their value comes from taking care of other people. They develop "other esteem"—the value they get from caring for others—rather than self-esteem. They are playing a role. They disconnect from their authentic self and from the place of self-love.

When these children become adults, they will enter into relationships limited by the role imprinted on them as falsely empowered children. As adults they feel like gods when they are taking care of other people. They feel they must do the right thing—that they must always appear to be good. They are often very successful people, but they have to be careful always to succeed and to appear good. They have to shut down their spontaneity in order to act always according to what they consider a plan for effective success. They were never allowed to be children, and, unless they change, they will never feel the joy of spontaneity.

Eventually their need to be mature becomes a burden, and they resent their godlike role. But for them it is an almost impossibly hard role to abandon. Their parents praised them for the role. Now their grown-up friends and colleagues do the same. They need the praise.

They have needed it ever since their parents made role playing a requirement of belonging to the family system. These Heroes and Heroines are the last people to get help. They reject anyone who tries to help them. They develop a profound sense of emptiness and boredom. They will seek intensity in order to overcome this deadness and often become risk takers, indulging in such things as secret sexual promiscuity, daredevil sports, and powerful stimulant drugs. On the surface of their lives there is the highly praised career and the good deeds. Its underbelly is a desperate and often immoral attempt to find vitality, which, if the community knew about it, would bring them disaster.

Sometimes falsely empowered children are smart enough and have experienced enough of the world to recognize that the parents who bestowed upon them the false power are very faulted people themselves. Hearing from their parents that they were the best was patently false. They come to realize that they have received the authority for their power from a false source. This realization is tremendously shaming and will often make them feel worthless, but these bouts of worthlessness are countered with returns to their role as Hero or Heroine. They become, in a way, the worthless Hero or Heroine. Stimulated by the drive of their false empowerment, they often achieve wonderful things. Shamed by the recognition that their virtues were falsely bestowed, they are unable to enjoy their true accomplishments. They can usually avoid being shamed by their community, but they cannot avoid being shamed from within.

Under *disempowering* abuse, children are shamed by the parents, either covertly or overtly. Covert shaming happens when children are neglected or abandoned. Stressed parents, aggravated by life into feeling that they do not have time to parent the children, turn their back on them. These children view their "inadequacy" (unworthiness of love), not as the result of septic acts of their parents, but as a general deficiency of their own whole being. The parents do not have to say anything. The message the children receive is that they are worthless—not even worth their parents' attention. The role assigned to these children is the Lost Child.

These covertly shamed children will lead a life of hiding out. They spend time getting high on fantasy, reading books, going to movies, being alone, being spaced out. They believe that they are inherently defective and start to shut the self down or to "disappear" themselves. In the place of the real self they invent a self that is designed to be "good" so as to get the parents' attention. Their "goodness" often goes under the guise of perfectionism. At the same time that these children are earning their value by being perfect, they are filled with the dread of being worthless. The sense of self is lost and, instead, they become defective souls going through life trying to keep their worthlessness from being discovered by others.

Overt disempowerment or overt shaming happens when children are blatantly pointed at and told that they are stupid or worthless in some way. This is probably the most deeply wounding form of trauma, leaving children with an inherent sense of defectiveness.

One form of trauma is both falsely empowering and disempowering at the same time. The message the parents are sending to the child is that he or she is very good at being very bad. This is seen in the role of the family Scapegoat. The child becomes the repository of all the bad thoughts and feelings the parents do not want to acknowledge about themselves. Ironically, in order to stay attached, even if it means continuous shaming, the child repeats the bad behavior and suffers the same consequence. In the concept of "being very good at being very bad," the "very good" part falsely empowers this child, while the "very bad" part disempowers the child at the same time. As adults, Scapegoats will spend a lifetime taking value from behaving badly and then suffering the shame directed their way by those whom they have offended.

In each of these kinds of childhood trauma—false empowerment, disempowerment, and the combination of the two—the authentic self of the child is devastated. Never having learned the concept of inherent worth because of the false roles assigned to them by their needy parents, these children have never learned to esteem from within.

According to the kind of abuse, the neglected or abandoned child becomes the Lost Child; the falsely empowered child plays the role of Hero or Heroine; and the covertly abused and falsely empowered child becomes the Scapegoat. The adaptive survival roles of Lost Child, Hero or Heroine, and Scapegoat inappropriately persist into adulthood, where they become adult actors plagued by self-centered fear, the pain of poor relationships, and an aching lack of intimacy.

If in life we can learn to identify the internal voices of our wounding that get provoked in relationships and to sabotage them, we can reclaim our true selves and behave more maturely in our relationships. Only then we will stand a chance at successful relationships and the gift of intimacy.

3
PERFECTLY IMPERFECT
The Authentic Child

And not in utter nakedness,
But trailing clouds of glory do we come
From God, who is our home:
Heaven lies about us in our infancy!
    —William Wordsworth,
        "Ode: Intimations of Immortality"

In my professional life I am close to pain and personal tragedy all the time, and I know pain and personal tragedy from my own childhood. But I believe that this pain is a declension from our birthright—in religious language it would be called a "fall from grace."

Despite what I know about childhood abuse and the pain of prolonged childhood, I do not have a tragic sense of human destiny. I have learned just the opposite—that an abiding sense of joy accompanies emotional well-being, and I believe that this joy is our natural inheritance. I believe that this joyful sense of rightness can be regained, that we can be reborn. As adults, we can experience this rebirth, and this recovery of our inherent worth can be learned in an orderly and rational way.

In her classic book *The Drama of the Gifted Child*, psychotherapist Alice Miller writes that when she used the word "gifted" in her title, she "had in mind neither children who receive high grades in school nor children talented in a special way. [She] simply meant all of us who have survived an abusive childhood thanks to an ability to adapt even to unspeakable cruelty by becoming numb. . . . Without this 'gift,' offered us by nature, we would not have survived."

If no parent is perfect, neither is any child: to emerge healthy from childhood is an act of recovery—not only from Alice Miller's "numbness"—but from keenly felt inadequacy and pain. It may sound like a contradiction in terms, but we recover our innocence through reeducation: we regain knowledge of our inherent worth; we learn to accommodate to our perfect imperfection.

The remembrance of our perfectly imperfect humanity is the bedrock on which the spirituality of recovery rests. Human beings have their limitations, but these limitations are not faults; they simply are part of the given truth about humans. If we learn to despise ourselves for being limited humans, we lose contact with the prime spiritual truth of our reality: that we are not perfect and that it is all right.

There is an authentic self. We are born with it. Under the influence of immature parenting, we lose contact with it. As children warped into shape by immature parenting, we get shamed about who we are. That shame gets bound to our experience of self. When we are "ourselves," we will have a shame attack, and in that attack we feel worthless. Spontaneity is frightening for us; it triggers shame attacks, bringing us back to our feeling of worthlessness. We wall in and shut down. Over the years, we become cautious in what we say and do. We lose contact with our authentic self. Rediscovery of the authentic self is what recovery is all about. (The etymology of "authentic" from its classical Greek root is true to the way I understand what the authentic self is. *Authentikos* derives from *authentes*, which means "author." The antonym of "authentic" is "counterfeit.")

There are five essential attributes of the authentic child that center around inherent worth. The attributes of childhood authenticity, connected to inherent worth like the spokes on a wheel, are *vulnerability, nascent reason, dependence, appropriate immaturity,* and *exuberant energy.* The mature, self-esteeming parent guides the child to the proper expression and development of each one of these attributes of the authentic child. The parent will be nurturing in the child what I call "boundaries." Boundaries are the psychological points of passage through which, on one hand, we express the truth of ourselves and, on the other, the information sent our way flows to us when we are in relationship. When our boundaries are functioning properly, what we express about ourselves respectfully communicates the truth of our emotions and ideas, and what we let in to our hearts and minds is relevant only to the emotions and ideas we hold to be true about ourselves. The requirement for healthy boundaries is self-esteem or inherent worth, the inculcation of which is the central job of parenting. The subject of boundaries will be discussed in dramatic detail in Chapter 9.

Inherent worth is often sabotaged by stressed-out parents who, while concerned primarily with meeting their own needs, silence their children for expressing their authentic selves. When they attack the children for displaying an essential attribute of their humanity, they make those children allergic to their true selves.

Let's imagine such abuse around the attribute of *exuberant energy.* The stressed parent, irritated by the child's exuberance and curiosity, shames the child into silence. The child gets the idea that being energetic and curious is something that makes her defective. The parent is implying that the child's energy is causing the parent damage. The child learns that to display her authentic self reveals her defectiveness, and she will have a strong reason to go into hiding. Paradoxically, one of the ways she will go into hiding is to become "perfect," matching her behavior to her anxious understanding of what her parent would ideally like her to be. Behind this mask of perfection hides her now suffocated authenticity.

Mature parents acknowledge the value of their children's energy and curiosity but explain that high energy has an effect on others. It is normal to have this energy, but it is in everyone's interest to contain it, so that someone else's personal boundaries are not being assaulted. Mature parents teach their children about relationship, adding to the children's sense of self *the sense of self in relationship.*

Let us consider the kind of parenting that must take into account the child's attribute of *vulnerability.* The child is not emotionally or physically strong enough to protect himself. If the parent does not provide that protection, either through neglect or active hostility, the child will learn that living is a dangerous proposition and his fear is appropriate. He develops his own system of protection to keep him safe from the harmful world. Because he must completely protect himself in order to survive, he creates a boundary in the form of walls. These walls defend him by blocking out the approach of other human beings. He anticipates that if he does not block out other human beings, he will be harmed, even annihilated. The system of walls blocks intimacy and is nonrelational, even though the child may appear to be relational by using various forms of superficial courtesies.

Let me point out here that when I use the term "boundaries," I am referring to a mature and functional use of the psychological energies by which we express and protect our sense of our true self when we are in relationship. In this functional sense, then, all exercise of our boundaries is good. Boundaries act like filters, allowing to come in and go out only those things that are appropriate to our psychological health, to the truth of who we are. Boundary failure takes two forms. Either there are no boundaries at all, in which case the integrity of the self is spewed away, or the boundaries have solidified into walls that permit nothing in or out. When there is no give and take, relationship is not possible. With that understood, having a "wall for a boundary" is a boundary failure.

One of the walls that the child might develop is the wall of fear. The child stays distant from others, because he has learned that closeness means to be injured. He has learned this reaction from his parents, who have not protected him from his environment, most often from the abusive parent himself, who, for example, might be a rager. In the face of his parent's rage, the child learns that if he tries to get close, he will be wounded. In an effort to survive, he will start distancing from the parent—not listening, not talking, staying away. The child is learning that to be relational is to risk annihilation.

At the same time that the unprotected child is learning about walls for boundaries, he is learning about boundaryless behavior as well. In the example of the raging parent, the child becomes familiar with and learns the boundaryless behavior of rage. This child will take on two dysfunctional boundary capabilities: he will distance with walls and he will go boundaryless, emulating the example of his raging parent. As he experiences his emotions, he goes boundaryless and releases that emotion in a way that assaults other people's personal boundaries. He has become an "offender," driving people away from him, isolating himself from intimacy with others just as effectively as he did with his system of walls.

Let us consider the developmental issues relevant to the authentic child's attribute of *dependency*. The child at first must depend on her parents to take care of her. In time, the parents' job becomes teaching the child to care for herself. When functional, mature parents take care of the child's dependent needs, they do so in a way that does not injure the child. A parent will be with the infant or very young child almost constantly and will respond immediately to the child's cries. He or she will pick her up and find out why she is crying, if she is hungry, or if she is too hot in her clothing, and so on. The parent will immediately attend to this, so that the child is kept comfortable. The idea that comes through to the child from this quick and constant care is that she has inherent worth. As the child grows, functional, mature parents will teach the child to do these things for herself. When the child is capable of doing these things for herself, the parents release these responsibilities to the child, but continue on in a supervisory role. The child has learned to care for the self and also understands that it is okay to get help from other people, that there is no shame or guilt attached to asking for assistance. The parents are teaching the child the very important lesson of *interdependence,* which is at the heart of mature relationality.

As the child continues to mature, the parents ask the child to become responsible for taking care of certain things that have to do with the family itself, such as washing the dishes or mowing the lawn. The child learns that she has a responsibility to be helpful to other people relationally. This is a form of being interdependent. She is learning a deep relational skill. Her mature parents have taught her that she has inherent worth; that she has responsibility for self-care, but that it is all right to ask for help; and that it is part of her responsibility to be helpful to other people.

With regard to her responsibility to be helpful to others, a mature parent will not ask too much from the child, so that the child does not get the idea that her job is to be a caretaker of others. She learns to allow others to be responsible and does not volunteer to take over what they should be doing themselves.

If parents are immature in regard to the child's attribute of dependency, they will turn their back by refusing to care for the child or by minimally caring for her. They may be caught up in their own concerns, whether business, stress, sports, gossip, sex, or substance abuse. The child's needs go unattended. The child wants and needs help, but gets little or, in the case of abandonment, none at all.

The child will learn to feel that she is not worthy of a caring relationship. The fault lies not with the child but with the parent, but because the nature of children is to be self centered, the child turns the parents' neglect into an indictment of herself. The child thinks that she is defective because she is not being taken care of. It is curious that by assigning herself responsibility for what is going on in terms of neglect, she gains the illusion of control and mitigates her own fear.

The child not only makes up the idea that there is something terribly wrong with her but experiences pain and fear, which teaches her that she is not able to take care of herself. She emerges into the adult world believing a lie that makes her feel overly dependent. She will look for others to take care of her.

To the people to whom she wants to relate she presents herself as a needy character, similar in her neediness to a child. Since other adults are likely to be looking to be relational with other adults, she is doomed to disappoint anyone who is looking for her to act self-sufficiently. Her partners resent having to take care of her and will distance from her. Their dropping her reinforces her idea that there is something wrong with her—that she is defective.

The other thing that immature parents do related to dependency is to appear to be taking care of the child's needs while their covert motive is to get her to care for them. Relationally what the child learns from being used this way is that it is her duty to take care of other people. Taking care of the parent drains energy from her and lessens her ability to get her own needs met.

For example, a mother who has been abandoned by her husband asks the daughter to parent her younger siblings. The mother needs time to make a life in the world and take care of her own needs. When the daughter spends her energies in performing the role of mother to her siblings and emotional support to her mother, she is drained of childhood energy. She learns that to be relational is enervating. She has no time to focus on her own issues.

Such individuals emerge in the adult world with a poor understanding of self-care, because they have learned that they have no right to ask others to care for their needs. They become "antidependent." They may take care of some of their own needs and wants, but their focus will be on others, and they emerge as caregivers who neglect their own needs.

People who cannot provide for their own needs because they have given themselves over totally to providing for others' needs are not being relational. By denying that they have needs, they take from their partner the ability to be interdependent as a giver as well as a receiver. The servitude of wantless and needless individuals appears spiritless, coming from those who have abandoned a sense of their own needs and wants. Such people are likely to be resented, despite the apparent goodwill of their giving, because their partner will feel that he or she is being manipulated into providing something the giver needs but will not express. The recipient will feel an obligation to be grateful, but senses the gift came from a place of dis-ease.

Nascent reason, or the incipient capacity to recognize the truth, is another attribute of the authentic child. All human children have the seed, or "chip," of reason—what the Greek philosophers called the *logos.* Their minds, properly nourished, will learn to tell the difference between truth and error; to distinguish relevant from irrelevant data; to see common denominators or analogies in complex data; and to tell what makes for success and what makes for failure in the ordinary tasks of life.

Immature parents may feel discomfort when a child first begins to identify his truth. For example, a child may see his father lying face down on the living-room rug, smelling of alcohol, with a whiskey bottle at his side. He runs to find his mother and tells her that Daddy is passed out in the living room. The child asks if Daddy is drunk. Mother's abashed reply is that he is not drunk, that he is just taking a nap. She brushes the child off by telling him to go outside and play. What happens to this child over a period of time in which such denials of truth have been repeated is that he will begin to doubt his own perception. In his natural self-centeredness, the child will make up the idea that he is incapable of knowing what is true and what is not. As he emerges into adult life, he will have a hard time owning his own reality. He will always live in reaction to other people's assessments of what is going on, thinking them superior to his own defective judgments. He pays little or no attention to his own mind.

People who doubt their own truth can never be real to their partner. They are always watching the partner so that they can adapt to the partner's evaluation of the truth. "No, tell me what you think of the situation," is a favorite reply. They become who they think the partner needs them to be. Their real self never turns up in the relationship, and the partner begins to feel that they are isolated from one another—indeed, that the partner is being left alone for want of an authentic presence to relate to.

A variation on the theme of parental abuse in the attribute of reason occurs when the parent allows the child's misapprehensions to go uncorrected. The parent never challenges the child and does not help him to think clearly. Perhaps the child has told his mother that the reason he hates school is that the teacher is always favoring the rich kids in the class. The mother backs up her son's excuse, perhaps mirroring her own resentment when she herself was struggling at school. "You are right, Tommy. Never trust the rich kids. They don't know a damn thing. It's people like us who really know what's going on." This child grows up confident in his delusion. He feels and acts as if he knows it all. When he enters a relationship, he cannot hear a competing opinion from his partner. He is disrespectful and intolerant. He becomes an offender—demeaning his partner's own right to express his or her truth.

When parents are being mature with their children concerning the authentic attribute of nascent reason, they spend a lot of time listening and supporting their children in expressing their thoughts and feelings and in giving them time and confidence to tell what is going on in their minds. When parents hear their children engaged in misapprehension, they offer the children a palatable rendition of reality according to logic and experience. Mature parents can do this without shaming the children into thinking that their own thinking processes are defective.

These children, confident of their ability to learn the truth, benefit not only from what they learn but from the process itself. They learn that the discovery of the truth includes making mistakes and being fooled. They learn not to be frightened or demeaned by making errors in the open-minded pursuit of evidence and truth. In relationships they are unafraid to express the truth as they see it and to be guided by the truth when they hear it from their partners. This ability to hear the truth and to be changed by it is a lesson in humility.

Mature parents have taught children that not knowing it all is not shameful. As the children own their truth in relationship and their partners challenge this truth, they will be able to hang on to their own truth while examining what they are being told. They will have developed the key ability to change their mind without a sense of defectiveness.

The fifth attribute of the authentic child is *appropriate immatu-*

rity. A child should feel comfortable acting her real age. She should not feel the need for power she does not yet own or for wisdom and judgment she does not yet have. At six she should not be expected to have the complexity and strength of a twelve-year-old. At fourteen, she must not seek to please by being as needy and undisciplined as a six-year-old.

An immature parent will praise a young girl by saying that she is only eight years old, but by the responsible way she acts you would think that she was fourteen. The parent has connived to create in the daughter an inappropriate maturity, so that the child can prematurely provide the parent with comfort. The parent is asking the daughter to take care of the parent. The child is never allowed to have a childhood.

In her effort to be mature, the child has aimed at finding her place in the family system. The security she has gained by controlling her spontaneity, however, has required that she deny herself freedom to be real. She winds up a person who is distanced from the self by severely containing the natural energy and ebullience associated with her true age. She does not know who she really is. In adult relationships, she will try to control herself and others. Her need to be in control is out of control.

Controllers give the message to their partners that the partners do not have the right to be who they are. Who the partner *is* is wrong. To their partners these people who are "out of control with being in control" will be shaming and troublesome.

Parents immature in regard to the attribute of appropriate immaturity may encourage a child to behave younger than her years. When a ten-year-old is having a temper tantrum in the way a two-year-old would, the parents indulge the infantile outpouring, appearing to get from it something like the reward a parent gets in the first years of a child's life when the child is totally helpless and dependent and the parent the guarantor of life. If the parent continues to seek this reward for being the parent of an infant beyond the time when the child is infantile, the parent can inflict severe damage. The child is encouraged to behave without containment. She emerges into adulthood with damaged capacities to contain her emotions or appetites. She is the kind of adult who does whatever she feels like doing. She is "in control of being out of control"—establishing her leverage in relationships on the lesson learned in childhood—that she is entitled to express herself without age-appropriate containment. One cannot have a relationship with a person like this. All one can do is step out of her way. People who have tried to have relationships with the out-of-control appetites of addicts have painfully learned this lesson.

Mature parents will know what to expect at each developmental stage. They will carefully allow children to act their age, and when they fail to act their age, the parents will confront the children along with an explanation and a description of the consequences of continuing to act inappropriately. Children learn that they cannot do just what they want to do, that there is always an expectation to act their age. Children are given information and instructions about appropriate maturity levels and literally receive support in growing up. As adults they will be able to distinguish between immature and mature behavior.

Because they know they have to act like adults, they provide their partner with the experience of having to deal with another adult, instead of slipping back and forth between adult and child states. If such stability is absent, partners will never be secure about whom they are facing and will sadly but wisely withdraw from such a relationship.

The manner in which the attributes of the authentic child have been nurtured molds the psyche of the adults the children will be-

come. In each of the child's attributes there is a road that leads more
to health than to dysfunction and a road that leads more to dysfunction than to health. The road children take will be irresistibly
mapped out by the conversations their parents or caregivers have
implanted in their heads. They become the tapes that roll in their
heart and brain even when they have become adults and think that
they have left childhood behind. What is certain is that children
learn to be relational with other people from being relational with
their caregivers—mainly with their parents.

As children develop language and listen to the language of the
parents, they begin to form a sense of who they are. They hear the
voice of their authentic self as well as the voices of their caregivers. If
the voices of the caregivers are at odds with the voice of the children's authentic self, the children adapt so that they begin to define
themselves under the inescapable influence of the abusive conversation their parents have with them. They may learn to doubt their
ability to know the truth. They may fear interdependence. They may
deny the exuberance of their youthful energy. They may develop
contempt for the opinion of others. They may think their job is to
care for others at the expense of self. In all of these distortions of the
authentic self they hear competing voices. They learn to have a conversation with self that makes it impossible for them to be authentic.

Recovery is about changing the conversation that has been
placed inside our heads by immature, abusive parenting. Understanding the content of these warring internal voices is crucial for us
and for our therapist. Before we have an inkling of what recovery is
about, we have no way of separating from the war inside our heads.
We think that the pain of the dissonance is what we call our "self"
and we let this dissonant self "act out."

As we take the first steps into recovery, we begin to understand
and to feel that the war between our inner voices can be mediated

by a mature, adult voice, which in celebrating our authenticity and our perfect imperfection gives us peace in our humanity. This discovery of the mature, adult voice inside ourselves is joyous. It returns us to a place of self-esteem and puts us in a position to enjoy healthy intimacy.

But before we can find this mature, adult voice, we have to learn about how and when the voices of our abusive childhood were implanted. The age at which they were implanted is important, because early trauma produces an ego state that is quite different from the one produced by later trauma.

Let us begin to examine how to begin throwing light into the recesses of childhood where the internal voices were first brought to life.

4

THE BIG PICTURE

*The truth as it is contained in the Christian revelation includes
the recognition that is neither possible for man to know the truth
fully nor to avoid pretending that he does.*
　　　　　　　—Reinhold Niebuhr
　　　　　　　(author of "The Serenity Prayer"),
　　　　　　　Beyond Tragedy

People who survive the trauma inflicted by a dysfunctional family
system develop complex ways to bear the pain and deny the truth of
the way they have been treated. As children they learn how to hide
and distort their authentic thoughts and feelings. They deny the
thoughts and emotions associated with traumatic events and the
caregivers who were responsible for perpetrating them. They mask
vulnerable emotions behind less vulnerable emotions. For example,
they may cover their fear with contempt or their pain with anger or
their sense of worthlessness with rage. These kinds of covering up
persist into adulthood, damaging their ability to have good relationships whenever old, unexamined traumatic memories are stirred up.
Recovery from childhood trauma begins with examining what actually happened to them as children, what they felt when it happened,
and how the resulting trauma distorted both their image of self and
their expectations for relationships.

The way we investigate our trauma history first requires that we identify our major caregivers, usually our parents, but the circle can widen to include a coach, doctor, priest, uncle, or aunt. We try to recollect what kind of emotion we associated with each. Were they "helpless," "loud," or "scary"? "Powerful," "meek," or "exhausted"? "Violent," "sexual," "angry," "silent," or "cold"? These short adjectives help us recall the emotions these caregivers created in us. From this information we can begin to make a map of how the caretakers related to one another. If Mom was "weak" and Dad was "angry," a picture of the family system begins to emerge from which we can learn by whom and how trauma was likely to be inflicted.

A key to recovery is that patients understand the big picture. The more they know about the process they are undergoing the better. I do not believe in the Freudian model of silent, invisible therapists who tell their patients nothing about the evolution of their problems. I have already written in Chapter 1 of the therapists whom I first met in treatment—how they related to their patients from the one-up stance and how this was as dysfunctional as the stance of their abject patients who were relating from the one-down position. For treatment to work, the relationship between therapist and patient must be empathic, not one of dominance and submission.

Trauma is the essential generator of fluctuations in self-esteem between one-up and one-down. If we are going to relate healthfully with our partners, we cannot listen or talk or express emotion maturely if either of us is one-up or one-down in relation to the other.

Since trauma is a chief cause of the fluctuations in self-esteem from one-up to one-down, we need to understand its etiology and the way it makes us unhealthy. Trauma is the chief generator of the problems we have in the core areas of our authentic selves: self-esteem, boundaries, reality, dependence, and moderation. When it affects our self-esteem, it can make us feel worthless; when it damages our boundaries, it can make us walled-in autocrats; when it affects our sense of reality, it can make us lose confidence in our ability to know the truth; when it damages our sense of healthy dependence, it can make us wantless or antidependent; when it damages our sense of moderation, it can make us believe that we are either bad or rebellious, rather than perfectly imperfect and human. When posttraumatic stress is awakened by something in our adult relationships, it not only damages our ability to be mature in one core area, but triggers dysfunction in all of them.

Determining the age at which people first received a traumatic wound is crucial in their recovery. If trauma is inflicted on infants or children up to about five years old, they will not have enough maturity, logic, or language skills to make a complex defense or adaptation in order to protect themselves. Their pain remains largely unexpressed. When such kinds of early wounding are stirred up in adults, their reaction to them will likely drive them back into this early ego state, and they will feel overwhelmed, flooded, and dissociative. In terms of behavior with a partner, they will go boundaryless and one-down. They feel bad about themselves and become too dependent and chaotic.

Reactions to trauma inflicted at a later age, let us say six to seventeen, will also make adults under the influence of posttraumatic stress feel childish, but this childish state feels like an adult state to the grown-ups. Because the wounds were inflicted on the children when they had some maturity and language skills, they were capable of building an adaptation that effectively counterfeited maturity. An adapted adult state for most people *is* as far as they get: the child masquerading as a grown-up.

When wounds are stimulated in individuals who have been traumatized at this later stage of childhood, if they have undergone falsely empowering abuse, their behavior in relationships is to go back behind a wall. They become aggressive and feel "better than" their partners. If they have undergone disempowering abuse, they will become yielding. They will become enablers and be manipulative. This behavior is commonly called passive-aggressive.

The emotions we feel at the time when our childhood trauma was inflicted are of two kinds. First there are the emotions we feel empathicly for our parents. We know their source, and we know what they have made us feel. We are aware of what is going on. We may feel deeply, but our boundaries remain intact. If, for example, our mother is frightened, we may feel the energy of her fear and feel along with her. Her fear energy has been "carried" through the air and we have taken it in. This kind of empathy can cause us discomfort, but we are not so bewildered or overcome by it that we lose our sense of self.

The second form of "carried energy," however, takes a much more insidious path and can come close to annihilating us. It is a boundary violation and occurs when carried energy is hurled at us with such intensity that it pierces our protective boundary. In the case of carried shame, for example, instead of being a witness to a shameless act, we feel we are the shameful actor, and we go to a feeling state of worthlessness.

Carried shame is the energy radiated from a caregiver when he or she has acted shamelessly toward a child but has not acknowledged it, often hiding the shameless abusiveness behind a wall of anger. The shame from which the parent has detached floats out into the room, and we begin to suck it up and carry that shame as if it were our own. Unlike the result of experiencing less toxic empathic responses that fall short of boundary violations, we go into a state of worthlessness. We can no longer recognize that the shame belongs to the caregiver. We think it is our own. We feel out of control and crazy; the energy we are feeling doesn't match our thinking.

Other kinds of energies can be carried to the point of boundary violations that annihilate self-esteem; here we know no longer the source of our emotions, thinking that what was given to us from outside has really come up from our own identities: rage, for example. In extreme cases of having to face a raging caregiver we are no longer just empathic, meaning feeling the anger of the caregiver while knowing its external source. In the vicinity of someone who is raging, we take on the carried rage and are compelled to rage ourselves. The boundary between the initiator of the rage and our own being has been breached. Or if we are in the vicinity of someone who is handling pain inappropriately, let us say by stifling it, we can take on enough of that pain to feel not only it but also the hopelessness pain often inspires. We have lost sight of where the pain came from. Thinking it is in us, we feel the helplessness that pain inspires.

Carried energies, particularly carried shame, are boundary-violating poisons spewed into the lives of adults by the ghosts of arrested development. In an attempt to leach the poison out of carried shame, "chair work," in which an individual is guided to give back his or her carried shame to the parents who are its rightful owners, is a crucial therapeutic technique.

"Chair work" gets its name from the chair or chairs recovering individuals set out for the actors from their traumatic past. They invite these people into the room and pull up a seat at a comfortable distance from them. A full description of chair work in action appears in the Appendix, where it is undertaken with professional assistance. However, as readers will discover (Chapter 9), as recovering individuals learn about how to control the emotional effects of shame attacks and boundary failures, the principles of chair work can be self-applied in order that they become aware of their traumatic vulnerabilities. As they learn the nature of their trauma history and practice boundaries to contain the pain of their continuing effect on them, they are in effect doing chair work on themselves.

During chair work, the individuals center themselves and become very calm and quiet. They close their eyes and begin to concentrate on their own breathing. They will feel themselves in a light trance. They imagine bringing a parent into the room for a talk in which they tell the parent how they felt when the parent traumatized them. They tap into the emotions they felt as a child but could not express. During chair work, they will be able to release those feelings from their body in a kind of emotional detox from the effects of the trauma.

If people can identify and release their carried shame, they are less likely to be reactive to those who stir up analogies to their original wounding. If this trauma-induced emotional toxicity is not released, whenever they are trying to be relational with a person who reminds them of their original abuser, the full panoply of dysfunctional emotions connected to all their core areas will be released. They will be helplessly enthralled in a child state while trying to be a relational adult. In such a state they will not be capable of relationality. Their partners will suffer or flee.

As the patients talk to their imaginatively materialized parents, I listen for "childish" thinking around the abuse issues. Often, as adults, patients will continue to think as children about how they have been traumatized. I identify these child states to the patients, and we talk about how a more functional and mature way to deal with the issue can be activated. But while I am talking what amounts to mature common sense, I am searching for a more technical and less obvious clue as to how my patients' carried energies need to be treated. It is here that I try to find out at what age my patients received their wounding.

During a relationship in which the wounds of arrested development are stimulated, dysfunctional adults will revert to either one of two childhood states. One is the "wounded child" and the other is the "adapted wounded child." When the trauma is stimulated, adults will feel the age they were when the original trauma was inflicted. They will act as though they are experiencing the emotion as they did when they were the child's age.

The *wounded child* is the younger of the child states: from birth to about five. In this state, the child will engage in magical thinking. His ego is tender and vulnerable. He thinks mostly without the aid of logic. As the child matures, his magical thinking starts giving way to reason. At this stage the adapted wounded child comes into being. He usually is six to seventeen. He can understand what is dysfunctional in his family-of-origin system and can figure out who he needs to be in order to make the system work in a way that will placate his dysfunctional parents. The wounded child has learned some new tricks and has become the adapted wounded child. The adapted wounded child has learned to change himself in order to manage the family system, which provides him, from his point of view, with survival.

These two child states replicate the extremes of the symptoms we have referred to before when we were describing in Chapter 3 the skews to the authentic self occasioned by immature parenting. In the younger, wounded state, the child begins to have a sense of being worthless. He has no boundaries or conceptual or linguistic abilities to contain or protect him. He is dependent and out of control. He becomes dissociated and overwhelmed. In the older state, the adapted wounded child feels one-up, "better than," powerful. He has learned to hide what he is feeling and to manipulate to get what he wants. He is walled in and shut down. He focuses on other people rather than on self. He is uptight and controlling.

It is ironic that the ego state of the adapted wounded child is about as mature as traumatized individuals are ever going to get without help. I say ironic, because as adults these kinds of people pride themselves on their ability to be mature. Often, I refer to this state as the "adult wounded child," because the identity they think of as their true adult self is in fact none other than the adapted wounded child dragged dysfunctionally into adulthood.

When I first began to do family-of-origin interviews and chair work, I noticed that when my patients described the trouble they had in relationships, they were not describing what I thought of as adult behavior. They were describing a child state revived: wounded child or adapted wounded child. No wonder they were having relational problems. Their altercations would degenerate into what appeared to me to be two little kids fighting it out. Adult negotiation was almost entirely missing.

The patients' early wounding had become part of their personality, and it was the part of the self that was getting them into trouble relationally. When patients were doing chair work, I showed them that when they were talking to a parent, they were experiencing emotion that referred back to child states. When they were feeling worthless and vulnerable, they were in the wounded state. When they were feeling one-up and all-powerful, they were in the older wounded adapted state. Their trauma issues created the ego states that they continued to use in their adult relationships. How their abusive parents originally related to them was getting mixed up in their adult responses. If a partner stirred up traumatic associations, they would start to act toward that person as if he or she were the one who had originally traumatized them.

The voice of the adapted wounded child is what patients identify as the adult self. This voice is walled in and judgmental, controlling and perfectionist. That part of the self will actually *parent* other parts of the wounded child. The voice of this parent will sound like the voices of the abusive parents. It is a voice that attacks, neglects, and refuses to relate to them or a voice that indulges them and damages their boundaries. The voice of the adapted wounded child mimics the voice of the parental abuser, making them feel bad about themselves and robbing them of self-esteem.

In order to find a way to arrest this vicious cycle, I developed the concept of the *functional adult* who would get into the middle of the conversation between the dysfunctional extremes. It would speak from a truly adult perspective. I will speak more of this later, but for now let me say that moving to the center between the extremes is the result of boundary work, which gives us the gift of moderation, without which all our dysfunctions are ready to fire away at us from their polar extremes.

I developed the concept of this functional adult voice during work on the core issues of self-esteem, boundaries, reality, self-care, and moderation. In looking at the whole relational recovery process, I realized that in treating the core issues and helping patients to go to center, we would need to develop an adult ego state in which there was no longer any one-up or one-down; instead, there would be an assurance of being okay, of having inherent worth, and embracing perfect imperfection. In this state of moderation and balance the possibility of intimacy could be reclaimed, as properly functioning boundaries allowed them to communicate their truth and listen to the truth of their partner without defensive manipulation.

In relation to the core issue of boundaries, instead of having walls or no boundaries at all, they would develop a boundary halfway between, so that they could be intimate with others without being too vulnerable. Instead of defining the self as good or bad, they would learn to define the self as perfectly imperfect. Instead of being too dependent or taking care of others and refusing help, they would learn to be responsible for self-care and to be realistically interdependent. Instead of being immature and out of control or uptight and controlling, at the center they would find balance and proper containment.

In recovery we consciously move to this centered, healthy ego state where the voice of the functional adult carries the preponderance of the relational communication. *The voice of the functional adult interrupts the conversation between the adapted adult child and the wounded child.* The functional adult now parents both those ego states by affirming their existence and also assures them that they now have a compassionate and mature parent to care for them. They do not have to fight for survival by abandoning their authenticity. Finally, they are in safe hands.

5

PHYSICAL INTIMACY

A Difficult Balance

I felt all flushed with fever
Embarrassed by the crowd.
I felt he found my letters
And read each one out loud.
I prayed that he would finish
But he just kept right on
Strumming my pain with his fingers
Singing my life with his words . . .
Killing me softly with his song.
—Roberta Flack

Having a good relationship is such a tricky business—this business of sharing truth with another, of talking and listening. The voices of our falsely empowered and disempowered childhoods still fight for a place in the script. They try to take over our vocal cords when we seek to share our adult truths. They want to sabotage our maturity and drag us back to the adapted or wounded dysfunction of the past. They try to make us take on the familiar role of Mama's Boy, Scapegoat, Lost Child, Hero or Heroine, Surrogate Partner, Surrogate Parent, or Family Counselor. The emotions this internecine strife provokes in us are what we feel in our relationships. And unless we know anything about trauma and recovery, we think these feelings are normal—just the way things are in a tough world.

It takes authentic self-esteem to give those abusive voices closure. When they are silenced or under control, relationships happen. Then we receive communication from our partners without the shame, fear, or panic that drives old voices to command us to attack, defend, or flee. From this place of self-esteem, we present our truth with love, or at a minimum with respect, for our partner.

People in relationship communicate their authentic selves to one another. When they seek intimacy, they are neither hostile nor defensive; when their partners seek intimacy from them, they are neither walled off nor resentful.

The currencies with which we share intimacy are our bodies, emotions, and thoughts. We give off energy from these sources and we receive them. When these energies are sent our way and we are receiving, we must choose to accommodate only the energies and truths that fit us.

For example, let us say your partner becomes angry with you because you do not want to go to a party that night. He says you are selfish for not wanting to go and all you ever think about is your own convenience. He says you do not love him. He not only says it, but perhaps he shouts it. If none of what he has said to you is true, if what you said about needing time alone is true, you must keep your partner's inappropriate energies and thoughts at a distance. You must do so, but in a way that is respectful of him. This discipline gives spiritual substance to the old concept of "not taking things personally." If you have respect for him, you will know that he is caught in up in some emotional bind that keeps him from seeing your truth. Something is wrong with his emotional state. He has a problem, and so does the relationship. You will want to help him for the sake of the relationship. Your self-esteem will be untouched.

You do not dismiss what is being shared with you. Instead, you recognize that the energy and misapprehension that your partner directed at you do not fit you. Your interest in coming to an understanding is so that the two of you can be intimate—so that you can both know the truth of what you are feeling and thinking.

A lack of *containment* is often at the center of troubled relationships. When someone directs emotion and thought at us and also when we are directing emotion and thought at another, we will become dysfunctional in either direction if we cannot properly contain our energies behind healthy boundaries. Let us say you want the girl you have just met and been attracted to to feel strongly about you. You tell her she's the most beautiful creature God ever created. You tell her you are bowled over and that no one else but she matters. She has become the center of your universe. This blast of energy, rather than pleasing your girlfriend, scares her. She thinks you may be crazy. After all, you hardly know one another, she thinks. She withdraws behind a wall.

When we become boundaryless, we allow in too much from another person or send out too much from ourselves. We may be too loud, too sexual, too emotional, or too overwhelming with our opinions or learning. When we are sending out too much stuff and bombarding our partner, she becomes vulnerable, victimized, resentful, and miserable. We have broken through her safety zone and caused her discomfort and pain.

On the other hand, when there is too much containment, we protect the self so carefully that nothing reaches us. We have constructed walls for boundaries and made ourselves invulnerable. Your partner might tell you he cannot trust you. You are unmoved. He touches you affectionately, and you have no reaction. He shares his opinions with you, and you seem not to have heard. You have shut down and stepped out of relationship. Without outside intervention, such as seeing a therapist, there is no possibility of change. With walls for boundaries, there is no such thing as a relationship. Intimacy has been denied.

Boundary dysfunction is experienced either as walls for boundaries or boundaryless excess; these are the extremes between which healthy boundaries operate. Like the functional adult I described in Chapter 4, who would get into the middle of the conversation between the dysfunctional extremes of the abused child, healthy boundary practice establishes the middle ground between our feeling too vulnerable and feeling invulnerable, between wanting to express too much and not wanting to express anything at all. A healthy boundary creates *controlled vulnerability.*

Controlled vulnerability keeps us open enough so that our partners can know us, but it defends us from destructive incoming energy. When we practice controlled vulnerability, we protect our partners from the unloving or disrespectful energies we have the potential as perfectly imperfect human beings to discharge. At the same time, we defend our authentic selves from the unloving or disrespectful energies for which we ourselves might get targeted.

To achieve controlled vulnerability one needs healthy boundaries. There are two kinds of boundaries that relate to physical and sexual contact or sharing. One refers to nonsexual closeness and touching and is called the *external physical boundary,* and the other is about sexuality and is called the *external sexual boundary.*

There are also internal boundaries that we use when we share ideas and emotions. To function intimately in relationship, we work both our external physical and sexual boundaries and our internal boundaries of mind and emotion.

Physical boundaries become relevant when we approach someone with the intention of getting physically close or when we invite someone to be physically close to us. These kinds of nonsexual approaches and invitations are in the realm of the *affectionate*. We may say good night to our hostess by leaning forward with the intention of kissing her cheek. Or she might take a step closer to us and incline her head forward, inviting us to kiss her cheek. Generally, whether being approached affectionately or approaching affectionately, we relax.

Affectionate approaches require controlled containment, because it is abusive to engage others in physical intimacy, even if it is nonsexual, without some sort of permission from them. Seeking permission is an act of respect and love and centers us in the truth of our wanting to be physically intimate with another. Many of us do not recognize that we are seeking intimacy. And some of us when we do something like kiss the cheek of the hostess are in fact not seeking intimacy, even if we mimic it. Maybe we are faking affection to hide the fact that we had a terrible time at the party. Sometimes we might be grandstanding, trying to go one-up with our display of graciousness. Sometimes we are being bullies, taking physical liberties so disguised by convention that their origin in sexual aggression is successfully camouflaged. But if we genuinely want to be affectionate, we will know the truth of our desire for intimacy and take responsibility for it. Intimacy is a serious transaction that requires agreement from both parties. If we want to kiss our hostess on the cheek, we might say, "May I give you a kiss?" When she says yes, the reward is warm relaxation. If she says no, how interesting!

The receiver of affection must practice containment also. As the other person approaches us, we should think of containing his affectionate offer so that what is offered matches what fits us. I know of a drunk who thought it was all right to rub his loins against his hostess's crotch as he said thanks for the party. By not keeping him at a distance and by not expressing her shame and anger, this woman suffered remorse, and the painful scene attacked her self-esteem for many days.

Protecting yourself and evaluating the content of an incoming offer is an act of self-esteem. You are centering on the truth of who you are and the kind of physical intimacy that fits your authentic feelings.

There is a boundary statement that sets up this particular transaction and it is *"I have a right to decide who touches me and who does not."* You have a right to control how close another gets to stand to you and whether they get to touch you and your private property—like your mail, phone messages, photographs, and diary. This boundary allows you to sort through a physical approach and make a decision about how vulnerable you choose to be.

The external physical boundary gives us the power to determine just how another person is going to be intimate with us. This is self-protection. In the act of containing the affectionate intimacy being offered we evaluate the details of what is coming our way and decide what we are going to allow. Because we are healthy, we are going to be open to only true and respectful information. Our expectation of receiving such true and respectful information pays the same spiritual compliment that we pay our self. Healthy practice of the external physical boundary is, therefore, an act of self-love and recognition of the truth of what the other person intends.

"I have a right to decide who touches me and who does not" is one-half of the boundary statement. The other half is *"The same is true for you."*

Ground Rules for Avoiding External
Physical Boundary Violations

1. Don't stand in another's personal space without permission. Generally speaking, eighteen inches from a person's body is considered that person's own private space and shouldn't be entered without permission.

2. Don't touch a person without permission

3. Don't get into a person's belongings—purse, wallet, mail, etc.—or living space without permission.

4. Don't listen to a person's personal or phone conversations without permission.

5. Don't expose others to contagious illness when you know you are contagious.

6. Don't smoke around nonsmokers in an identified nonsmoking area.

Let us now consider the external sexual boundary. I have a responsibility as I am approaching somebody sexually to contain myself sexually in the interest of the comfort of the other person. This action involves the establishment of the external sexual boundary. The boundary statement that sets up the healthy exercise of the sexual motive is *"I have a right to control with whom, when, where, and how I am going to be sexual. And the same is true for you."*

If I concentrate on the first part, this boundary statement empowers me to make my own decision about whether to be sexual with someone, whether I like him or not, and, if I agree to be sexual, I still have the responsibility and the right to determine when, where, and how I want to do that. When I protect myself this way, I am performing an act of self-love. I am dealing with the truth of my sexual motive and my partner's.

Our external sexual boundary must be in place when someone is approaching us with sexual motives. We have to be respectful of what that person is saying to us about when, where, and how. We cannot just demand our way. As we are being physically or sexually intimate, we either signal our availability or discourage it, but with respect.

Ground Rules for Avoiding External Sexual Boundary Violations

1. Don't engage a person sexually without permission.

2. Don't insist on having your way sexually in the face of another's "no."

3. Don't demand unsafe sexual practices.

4. Don't expose others to sexual experience without permission.

5. Don't sexually shame another person.

When you have a functional boundary, you protect and contain yourself while remaining vulnerable enough for intimacy but not so vulnerable that you can be easily damaged. When you have a wall for a boundary, you block all intimacy and become invulnerable and, therefore, incapable of intimacy. When you have no boundary, you do not protect yourself from other people at all, so you get victimized a lot. With no boundary, you also do not contain yourself, so you regularly offend people.

The protective part of an external physical boundary could be a wall, but the containment part of the same external physical boundary could be nonexistent. Boundary systems are different from person to person, and their power in one area or weakness in another generates what kind of people we become in relationships.

External Physical and Sexual Boundary Architecture

Here are examples of the external physical and sexual boundaries when (1) the boundary system is intact, (2) when there is a wall, and (3) when there is no boundary. In each instance there is a protective part and a containment part.

EXTERNAL PHYSICAL PROTECTIVE BOUNDARY

1. The external physical boundary establishes distance and non-sexual touch. When the protective part of the external physical boundary is functioning properly, the individual decides who is going to touch him, how close he will permit other people to get to him, and whether he will permit them to touch his private property.

2. When the external physical protective boundary is a wall, the individual never lets anyone get near to her; nor does she permit anyone to touch her private property.

3. When the external physical protective boundary is nonexistent, the individual will let anyone get in his face or touch him physically, and he permits anyone to get into his private property without saying anything.

EXTERNAL PHYSICAL CONTAINMENT BOUNDARY

1. If the external physical containment boundary is functioning properly, a person will not get in someone's face or touch her or get into her personal things without permission.

2. When the external physical containment boundary is a wall, the individual never approaches another person to stand close or to touch, and others never get near his personal things.

3. When the external physical containment boundary is nonexistent, meaning the person has no self-containment at all, at his whim he will touch other people, get in their faces, and get into their private stuff without asking permission.

EXTERNAL SEXUAL PROTECTIVE BOUNDARY

1. When an individual's external sexual protective boundary is functioning properly, he decides who, when, where, and how someone is going to be sexual with him. As someone approaches him, he figures out if he wants to be sexual, and if he chooses to, he decides when, where, and how he will do that.

2. When an individual's external sexual protective boundary is a wall, he never responds to a sexual approach. He walls off from sexual approaches, acts as if they were not happening, and refuses to be sexual.

3. When an individual's external sexual protective boundary is nonexistent, he cannot say no to any sexual approach and is sexual with anyone who wants to be sexual with him.

EXTERNAL SEXUAL CONTAINMENT BOUNDARY

1. When an individual's external sexual containment boundary is functional, he always asks and gets permission before becoming sexual with his partner.

2. When an individual's external sexual containment boundary is a wall, he never makes sexual approaches to anyone.

3. When an individual does not have an external sexual containment boundary, he makes sexual advances without permission or in the face of the other person's refusal.

6

EMOTIONAL AND INTELLECTUAL INTIMACY

The More Difficult Balance

Let me not to the marriage of true minds
Admit impediments. Love is not love
Which alters when it alteration finds,
Or bends with the remover to remove.
O no, it is an ever-fixed mark
That looks on tempests and is never shaken . . .
　　　　　　　—William Shakespeare,
　　　　　　　　"Sonnet 116"

I have been discussing the external physical and sexual boundaries we exercise when we seek or receive physical intimacy—whether affectionate or sexual. Healthy behavior in the area of the external physical boundaries is an easier subject to approach than the boundary politics of internal intellectual and emotional intimacy, because the energies that excite our imaginations and emotions lie beneath the surface and mingle with the complex and obscure stories of our childhoods.

What we know about the truth is limited to what our individual perception of it is at any given moment. Telling the truth is our best guess about what is going on with our thoughts and emotions. Despite the subjectivity of our perceptions of what the truth is, if we do not act on the basis of what we genuinely believe it to be, our attempts at intimacy will fail. Truth's basis in individual perception is a good reason for us to own it with humility.

To be respectful and loving toward our partners, we want to be comfortable in front of them. Our partners, to be loving and respectful of us, also need to feel comfortable in front of us. When our boundaries enable us to communicate our truth and to receive truth without pain, fear, and anger, the conditions for comfort exist. Communication skills are so often taken for granted that we are blinded to how difficult communication is in relationships. Relationships require maturity and skill, and, fortunately, when we learn the skills, maturity follows. Boundary work is the most important tool in developing the kind of emotional communication that leads to intimacy in relationship.

The two boundaries we exercise when we are relating intimately in the areas of intellect and emotion are the *internal listening boundary* and the *internal talking boundary*. Almost all troubled relationships suffer from partners who have boundary failures that damage their ability to listen or talk without interference from their trauma histories. Our internal listening boundary protects us from the thought and emotions of our partners as they reach out for intimacy with us. We exercise our internal talking boundary in order to protect our partners as we reach out for intellectual and emotional intimacy with them.

When someone is talking to us and directing emotion our way, our internal listening boundary allows us to remain sensitive and engaged, while at the same time protected from painful, false, or irrelevant data and emotion. Exercising the listening boundary empowers us to sort through the ideas and emotions that are being directed at us, allowing inner access only to ideas and emotions that we deem appropriate. This selection process is controlled by what we know of our authentic self—by how intimate we are with our own truth. Our desire to protect our authenticity from damage is, therefore, self-esteeming—an act of self-love on the behalf of our authenticity.

In order to exercise the listening boundary, we cannot feel physically or sexually coerced. We are neither in someone's face, nor is he or she in ours. We need enough physical room between us to feel engaged but not so much that we become remote. We need room to sort and filter incoming intellectual and emotional energy. The distance from which we choose to communicate with our partners will differ with individuals, and we each have to agree that the distance is okay for us. If someone is too close to us, we respectfully say that we are going to take more space. We do not offend when we make this request. If we need more engagement, we say so and ask if we may move closer.

The next thing we have to do when we are exercising the internal listening boundary is to remind ourselves that the goal of our listening is to discover the emotional identity of the person who is talking to us. If we remain confident in our role of investigator, we will not wall out the other person because of distaste or fear of what we may learn, because if we do, our source of information disappears. If we remain self-assured in our investigative attentiveness, our alert receptivity will open up our partners so that they are likely to share intimately and reveal their true self, which is the goal of our investigation.

The third thing we must do is to remind ourselves not to be so open that we forfeit our ability to sort, filter, and reject. We have to determine if what we are hearing is true, untrue, or questionable.

When we hear words we believe to be true, we allow the information to get close to us. We permit ourselves to have feelings about what we are hearing, and we identify those feelings clearly. Is it anger or is it fear? Is it love or is it lust? Is it shame or is it guilt? Perhaps it is joy. It is surprising how many people cannot recognize when they are feeling joy. (So many of us think that only the relative highs yield joy that we fail to credit the joy in "mere" serenity). The distinctions are important and not always easy to make accurately.

If what we hear is not true, our boundary denies access to the false information and interrupts the process by which that information generates a feeling. We back off from personal intellectual and emotional responsibility for the falsehood and concentrate instead on what the falsehood tells us about the person who promulgated it. No matter if we disagree, we remain respectful, giving our partner the right to have whatever thoughts and emotions he or she is experiencing. We acknowledge that our partner believes in the truth of what is being said, and we remind ourselves that it is our partner's truth that we are discovering so that we can know him or her. In this process, we remain available to hear who our partner is but take in only what matches our truth. We do not take it personally that our partner has different ideas than we do.

It is not only thoughts that have to be evaluated for truth and admissibility. We need to be *physically* aware of the kind of emotional energy that is being emitted at us. Emotions come off the body in the form of energy. In the process called empathy we take another's energy into our bodies and feel (identify with) what that emotion is like for the other person. The listening boundary gives us time to identify the incoming emotion and decide with how much of it, if any, we will be empathic. We do not want to be overwhelmed with empathic energy; for in that case we lose contact with our true self.

If we are tired, for example, and the emotional signals from our partner call on us to expend a lot of empathic energy in order to join our partner at the same energy level, it is a good idea to back off. We might call a metaphorical time-out, making it clear that we are not prepared at the moment for such excitement. If we do not, we will exhaust ourselves, become resentful or perhaps remorseful when we only pretend to be playing the game, and then kick ourselves for having acted falsely.

We use the *internal talking boundary* when we approach our partner with our thoughts or emotions. We focus on containment so that our truth is neither explosive nor offensive. Our essential goal is to communicate our truth without manipulation, without inserting a covert agenda into the information we are sharing. Manipulation is controlling and toxic and destroys intimacy. We need to remind ourselves that we are talking to be known and not to control or to manipulate.

To tell the truth about how we feel, it is important to be clear. We tell about our experience in terms of what we saw, heard, tasted, felt on our skin, and so forth. We do not use adjectives that propagandize in favor of our desired effect. Here is an example of some emotional testimony from someone who is not using her internal talking boundary.

Mary wants to talk with John about something he has done to upset her. She says, "When I came into your *vile* little apartment, I saw that *bitch cuddling up* to you while you *blabbed* on the phone to your *stupid* mother. I knew you were up to *no good*." This approach is definitely not designed to get John in the right frame of mind to listen to what Mary may legitimately have to share with him about his behavior.

If she had said something like, "When I came into your apartment, I saw a woman standing close to you while you were talking to your mother. What I felt about that was that I was unimportant to you, and I felt pain and anger." If Mary had her internal talking boundary functioning, as she did in the second example, John could have shared his thoughts and feelings about what Mary just told him. In the second example, nothing that Mary said to John was controversial or in anyway deniable. She said that she entered the apartment, saw a woman standing near him while he talked to his mother, and that she then felt unimportant and felt pain and anger. If John uses his internal listening boundary, he will know that Mary made up something about what he did and became pained and angry. If he wants to be intimate with her, he will try to find out why she felt that way and what his part was in it.

Mary has shared her feelings and now John can share his emotions on hearing what she has told him. They both know there is a problem. They can focus their intellects and emotions on respectfully telling the truth in as clear and simple a way as possible. They contain their emotions, not overwhelming each other with contempt, rage, or fear. They do not infect the air. They tell the truth about self and, in so doing, love the self. They listen to truth and that is an act of love and respect for other. The communication between them is intimate, making love possible.

Intimacy, which discovers love in one human relationship, contains the model for its discovery in all human beings. Loving relationships discovered and preserved through the practice of boundaries require the conclusion that all human beings have inherent worth. It is always capable of being rediscovered, never capable of being destroyed. The source of that love is a Power greater than any self. To have that revealed is to be on the spiritual path.

Ground Rules for Avoiding Internal Listening and
Talking Boundary Violations

1. Don't imply by word or deed that another person is worthless. That is called shaming another person.

2. Don't yell or scream at another person.

3. Don't ridicule another person.

4. Don't lie.

5. Don't break a commitment for no reason.

6. Don't attempt to control or manipulate another person.

7. Don't be sarcastic while being intimate. The Greek etymology of "sarcastic" means "rending the flesh."

8. Don't interrupt.

Internal Listening and
Talking Boundary Architecture

Here are examples of the internal listening and talking boundaries when (1) the boundary system is intact, (2) when there is a wall, and (3) when there is no boundary.

INTERNAL LISTENING PROTECTIVE BOUNDARY

1. When an individual's internal listening protective boundary is functional, he filters what other people are saying and takes in only truth. He matches his truth against what he is hearing and takes in

only what is true for him. When what is being said is questionable or untrue, he keeps it out or does not react to it, letting it pass through him without effect.

2. When an individual has a wall for an internal listening protective boundary, he never listens to what the other person is trying to say to him, even if it is important.

3. When an individual has no internal listening protective boundary, he takes in everything the other person is saying, even when it does not match his truth, and is vulnerable to it all.

INTERNAL TALKING CONTAINMENT BOUNDARY

1. When an individual has a functional internal talking containment boundary, he concentrates on telling the truth in a respectful manner. He tries to be politic and diplomatic.

2. When an individual has a wall for an internal talking containment boundary, he never tells anyone what is important to him.

3. When an individual has no internal talking containment boundary at all, he says whatever comes to mind without monitoring whether it is true or not and doesn't care whether he is speaking respectfully.

7

THE BLAME GAME

*Speak not to me of blasphemy, man. Why I'd smite the sun if it
insulted me. For its doing that, then could'st I the other.*
— Herman Melville,
Captain Ahab in *Moby Dick*

Intimacy requires that we adjust our communicative energies in the
interests of our partner's comfort. We also require that our partner
adjust his or her communication in the interest of ours. This give
and take in the interest of intimacy and comfort demands from the
relationship commitment, loyalty, and cooperation.

It takes a while to work out the ground rules of intimacy, and we
have to be committed enough to the relationship to hang in there
while difficulties are being resolved. As they say in AA, "Don't leave
before the miracle happens."

We have to be loyal. Loyalty is about backing up your partner
when the partner is in conflict with someone else. The matter becomes complex if you do not agree with the position your partner is
taking, or if at the time that you are witnessing your partner's conflict, you and your partner are not getting along. You are tempted to
inflict pain on your partner by siding with the adversary. You are
certainly tempted to say what you think of your partner in front of
the adversary. Here is where diplomacy becomes important, and

diplomacy is part of the world of politics. We usually do not think of politics as an area for the practice of spirituality, but in intimate relationships it is.

When we share thoughts, body, or emotions, we have to make sure that we are caring for our long-term interests by being politic or diplomatic about what kinds of information we are willing to reveal. This kind of controlled intimacy is made possible by healthy boundary work.

We have to think carefully about exposing potentially harmful truths about our self, such as telling our intimate partner that we are siding with the adversary. Within relationships we must be diplomatic for the relationship and politic for the self. It would be neither politic nor diplomatic, for example, for a husband to tell his wife that he thinks her best friend is sexually attractive and that he has often thought about having sex with her. It would not be politic or diplomatic even if it were true. By not sharing that sort of information we are being politic for self and diplomatic for the relationship.

One sure-fire way to step out of diplomatic intimacy is to engage in the *blame game.* Blaming is a result of profound immaturity.

When we are infants, we are mostly a blank slate, what the philosophers call a *tabula rasa.* At this stage in our development, we depend on our parents to provide us with the feelings and behavioral routines that compose our personalities. Dependence at this stage in life is normal. When the dependence is prolonged into adulthood at the expense of a self that makes independent values and is emotionally self-generating, it becomes codependence and lies at the center of our adult emotional difficulties in relationships. Healthy boundaries enable us to work our side of the street and to stop blaming others for the way we feel. They allow us to be ourselves.

We stop blaming other people for what is going on physically or sexually with our bodies. We stop blaming other people for what we are thinking or feeling and what we have chosen to do or not to do.

The exercise of the talking boundary is useful in clarifying where our responsibility for our own feelings lies. Let us say that during a business meeting at which Peter is making an oral presentation, Susan pushes back from the table and leaves the room. Peter does not like this at all. If Peter has no skills in the exercise of boundaries and, therefore, of the talking boundary, he might confront Susan after the meeting and say something like, "When you set out to humiliate me in front of all those people by barging out of the room with not a thought to my feelings, you made me enraged and you made everyone think I was a laughingstock."

The fact is that Susan may have left to go the rest room and that the other members of the meeting thought that Peter's presentation was just splendid. Because the only truth we know is so conditioned by our own perception of it, our talking boundary, properly exercised, will limit us only to what is incontrovertible.

Peter might say, after the meeting and after placing himself at a comfortable distance from Susan (one that makes her feel comfortable also), "Susan, when you left the room when I was presenting my report to the group, what I made up about that was that I was not respected, and I felt shame, pain, and anger." Note that he has not told Susan that she made him feel any of these emotions. He told her that when she did what she did, he put his own interpretation on it and then had feelings about what he had made up. Only Peter could have generated the emotions he felt. Susan did not make him feel them. In fact, without changing Susan's actions at all, he might have had another kind of report to make: "Susan, when you left the room when I was presenting my report to the group, what I made up about that was that I was a threat to you, and I felt joy and pain. I felt joy, because I saw in your fear of me evidence of my power in the company, and I felt pain because I empathized with your pain." The two reports of his emotionality vary with Peter, not with Susan.

We also stop taking blame from other people for having made them feel the way they do. It is not appropriate to take the responsibility for what is happening to others' bodies, minds, and emotions or what they are choosing to do or not to do. Remember this the next time someone tells you, "You give me a headache." If you process that remark healthfully, you will recognize that that person has made up something about you that has made her have a particular feeling. So far you do not know what that feeling is. She probably does not know either. She calls the feeling "a headache." You will probably be interested in how she arrived at having a headache, but you will not take blame for having caused it.

The only exception to this rule is when we are in the presence of someone who has lost all containment and become an offender, one whose assault causes such direct damage that blame is obviously legitimate to assign to him or her. Except in a case like this, the place to look for the causes of our feelings is not in others, but in ourselves. Like Captain Ahab, whom I quoted in the epigraph to this chapter, we blame the white whale for all our difficulties and, like Ahab, we commit blasphemy against the self by surrendering moral responsibility to an outside agency.

Ground Rules for Avoiding the Blame Game

1. Don't blame others for what is going on with your body.

2. Don't blame others for what you are thinking.

3. Don't blame others for what you are feeling.

4. Don't blame others for the choices you make.

8

TALKING AND LISTENING BOUNDARIES

This chapter is practical. It may even sound like a self-help article from one of those glossy magazines. I have nothing against glossy magazines except for the fact that their self-help advice is usually absolutely obvious and completely useless. Such as when your husband is treating you badly, and you are advised to remember that he is "precious." Or when you feel the urge to spend money to make yourself feel better, and you are advised that money is not what is important; self-esteem is. Or when you want to lie in order to keep yourself from being embarrassed, and you are reminded that "Honesty is the best policy."

The fact is that we all want to be better, but most of us don't want to get better. It seems too hard or risky or bewildering. As a witty therapist once told me, "We forget that if we don't change direction, we'll wind up where we're headed."

We can take a long step forward in our search for spiritual peace if we learn the techniques by which we keep our talking and listening boundaries intact. If we do so and protect ourselves from inappropriate talk coming in at us (protected listening) and inappropriate talk coming out from us (contained talking), *we achieve an automatic balance that replicates truth and respect.* In that *artificially* created environment that is the gift of boundary work, the *real* thing comes into being. It's sort of like what they say in AA when they are pointing out that good feelings will follow good actions: "Fake it until you make it." Or as I said in the beginning of this book, it is the nature of the boundary system to create the experience of truth and respect.

The listening and talking boundaries do that for you. They will change your life from the inside. At first, the exercise of the talking and listening boundaries may seem "fake," in the sense that it is so different from our usual way of behaving in relationship that it doesn't seem genuine to us. The good news is that it will come to seem genuine, and when it does, you will achieve a true intimacy in relationships, which will have the additional immeasurable benefit of putting you on the spiritual path.

Ground Rules for Exercising the Internal Talking Boundary

1. Set your external physical boundary in order to be more comfortable as you talk.

2. Remind yourself not to blame.

3. Remind yourself you are sharing to be known, not to control or manipulate.

4. Remind yourself to moderate your emotions through breath work: breathe deeply when you are experiencing emotion.

5. State what happened or what you want to share without using words that are demeaning (report sensory input, what you saw, heard: "You play the television long and loud").

6. State what you believe or made up about what you stated in Rule 5 (thoughts: "What I made up about that was that you did not care about my comfort").

7. State how you feel or made yourself feel regarding what you said in Rule 6 (feelings: "And I made myself feel angry and I felt shame").

8. State what you did regarding your thoughts (stated in Rule 5) and your feelings (stated in Rule 6): "And I decided to talk to you about the way you handle the television set and the way I feel about that."

9. State how you would prefer things to be, if appropriate. If negotiation is required, start this process as follows: identify the problem; propose various solutions; choose one solution; and put the solution into action. Evaluate the results to see if further negotiation is necessary.

The very first thing you want to do before you talk to somebody is to set the distance you need between you and the other person in order to talk in a comfortable way. That is called setting your external physical boundary: it is the boundary that establishes a comfortable distance for you.

Bodily sensations can help you gauge the distance. If you are standing too close to someone when you begin to speak about an uncomfortable issue, your body may give you the sense that you want to tip or move back. You feel that if you started to talk, the words would be pushed back into your mouth. In contrast, if you were standing too far away, you might notice your body giving you the sensation that you want to move or incline forward. Your body is helping you determine a comfortable distance for the conversation.

For example, suppose Michelle is thinking about talking to her husband, Mark, about what she saw him doing with his ex-wife, and she knows that he doesn't want to hear about it and will likely be angry. She undoubtedly knows that she does not want to get too close to him. So she would think, not only about what she wants to say but about what she historically knows about his behavior when this subject is brought up, and choose her distance according to her feelings.

If she noticed that he was standing in their U-shaped kitchen with a counter on one side, her initial impulse might be to go out the back door and talk to him through the kitchen window. But that would be inappropriate. It would be better to stand on the other side of that counter, which would give them about six feet of separation. Then there would be that barrier between the two of them, so that Michelle could get closer if she wanted to, but not so close that she couldn't get the words out because she was feeling Mark's energy in her face.

This selection of her distance from her husband would be thought through in advance. Let us say that Michelle is six feet away from Mark behind the counter and he is standing at the stove. Rule 2 reminds her not to blame him for what she is thinking, for what she is feeling as a result of that thought, or for what she would like to do as a result of what she is thinking and feeling.

When she forms her sentences describing her thoughts or emotions or what she did or would like to do, she would not use the phrase "made me," as in "When you did that, you *made me* angry (sad, happy, hopeless)." For example, she should remind herself *not* to say, "When I saw you do that, what you made think or feel or do was this." We must always take responsibility for our own thoughts, observations, emotions, and behavior.

The third thing to do is at the heart of the boundary and is one of the most important things to concentrate on: you are talking to your partner to be known by him or her, *not* to try to control or manipulate. When most people are talking about a subject that is difficult for them, they have the urge to manipulate or control. They want to effect some sort of outcome as a result of what they are saying. You know that you are in that manipulative, controlling state of mind when you ask yourself the question "Am I saying this to my partner *so that* . . . ?" The words you want to pay attention to are the words "so that." If "so that" is in there, it means that you want a certain outcome and that you probably have some attachment to it.

If you discover that when you are talking you are using the manipulative "so that," you have to admit to yourself that you want the other to change behavior in some way and that you want a different outcome than what is going on. You also have to admit that to your partner. For example, Michelle might say,

"So listen, Mark, what I would like to do is share with you some observations, thoughts, and emotions I have about how you interacted with Nicole last week. Before I do that, what I want to share with you is that I'm really trying to control something here. I am quite attached to the outcome. I would really like you to change certain behavior, and I have a lot of attachment to that. I have to admit to that, because I really have to say to you that you have a right to be who you are, and that I don't have a right to control or manipulate you into who I want you to be. I want you to know that because there is some energy of attachment around what I am saying."

When you do make such a candid admission of the truth of what you were thinking and feeling, it enables you to let go of that attachment, with the understanding that your partner is a precious person who has a right to be who he or she is and that you have a right to share who you are. Though you would like your partner to be different, you do not have the right to tell your partner how to be on this planet. (An exception to the foregoing occurs in a boundary violation, for example, when someone physically, mentally, or verbally abuses you by means of a direct attack on your self-worth, often accompanied by screaming and name-calling.)

It is important not to allow the emotions you experience while you are talking to build and become too powerful. That is where Rule 4 comes in. Without breath work, the energy that is building in you starts to radiate and blast out toward your partner.

Rule 5 is to begin establishing your actual talking boundary. You state what you observed. Then you state what you say happened. I call this the sensory input: what you saw with your eyes, what you heard with your ears, what you smelled with your nose, what you tasted on your tongue, and what you physically felt on your skin. As Joe Friday used to say, "Just the facts."

You have to be very careful not to use any words that demean your partner or anyone else involved in any way. For example, if Michelle did this incorrectly in speaking to Mark, it would sound like this:

> "Last night you thoughtlessly came home late without calling me to tell me that you were going to be late. You barged through the front door like a rhino, slammed the door against the wall, and like a compete jerk you went to the bedroom without saying a word to me."

The words "rhino" and "jerk" are demeaning. Michelle needs to talk to Mark respectfully about his behavior.

"Last night you came home late. You promised me that you would call if you were going to be late, and you didn't. When you opened the door, you jerked it open and it slammed against the wall. Then, without saying a word or even looking at me, you walked through the kitchen, down the hall, into the bedroom."

In this last instance Michelle has not used words that refer to Mark as "less than" in any way. She was literally saying just what she observed without doing any editorializing.

The next thing Michelle would say is what she thought about Mark's behavior (Rule 6). Here is a dysfunctional response:

"You are insensitive, offensive, and self-centered."

A functional response would be

"Number one, you didn't follow through on an agreement we had, which was that you would call if you were going to be late. And what I think about that is that you have violated an agreement we had and were, therefore, offending me."

Michelle is not talking in a way that is demeaning to Mark. She is just stating what she thought.

The next thing Michelle would say comes under Rule 7. She would state what emotions she had regarding what she had just said in Rule 6, that is, about breaking an agreement and making up that he felt guilty about what he was doing the night before.

"I felt angry and afraid."

Note that in Rules 6 and 7 she did not say that "you made me" think or feel any of these things.

If Michelle had taken action on account of what she thought (Rule 8), she would say what she did about what she thought or observed:

"I called your office to see if you were still there, and I didn't get any answer."

Michelle wants different behavior from Mark, but she states it as a preference:

"In the future, if you are going to be late, I would prefer it if you would call me and let me know. And also I would prefer it if in the future that when you come home, you would acknowledge that I am there instead of saying nothing to me and just going to bed."

Michelle uses the word "prefer" because she does not have the right to control how Mark has to come home and what he has to say when he does.

Mark's breaking of the agreement to call when late is a boundary violation. When we make a commitment to somebody to do something and break it without any explanation, essentially we are in violation of that person's boundaries. Michelle could say on this issue:

"When you didn't follow through on what you had agreed to, I knew that was a boundary violation, and I really want you to stop making commitments and not following through, because it is abusive to me."

The main thing you want to concentrate on in maintaining a healthy talking boundary is containment—*respectful containment*—so that no blaming whatsoever comes out of your mouth. There should be no controlling or manipulating going on. And another thing on which you must concentrate is to not use condescending, patronizing, or sarcastic language that shames or demeans. Such language puts you into an abusive one-up position, which looks down on the other person, makes relationality impossible, and amounts to a self-esteem failure on your part—the failure of grandiosity.

Maintaining boundaries takes energy. It requires being alert and ready to put our boundary skills to work. Even though we may have had a fair amount of boundary practice, because we are perfectly imperfect human beings, the words of our partners will cause us to make up that we have been demeaned and we may feel pain, shame, anger, or fear. When we have generated these emotions as a result of becoming improperly vulnerable, we rely on a technique to reduce the emotion and to keep it from infecting the air, thereby making our partner a victim of our carried energies. What we want to do is "breathe them into submission." That is right. We take a deep, slow breath and imagine the emotion we are feeling as having a bodily presence right before our eyes. Then we breathe into it and let it go. We imagine it passing right through us like a ghost. This way, we keep the emotion from becoming toxic, floating out into the air, and infecting our partner.

When we breathe into the emotions we feel about what someone has said about us, we are learning a lesson in *humility*, and that lesson is that we are never totally free of our traumatic past; that will always have some traces our childhood abuse within us. We are not perfect, but we can be aware.

If we failed to contain ourselves and lashed out in resentment at an offense we made up we had received, we owe our partner amends. Exercising our talking boundary, we share with our partner the process by which his or her words, actions, and thoughts led us to go back along a path on which we made up painful emotions. We free our partner from blame. We take responsibility. It is a very spiritual moment. In such moments love and trust are kindled.

We might solace ourselves by reminding ourselves of our imperfect humanity. We might compliment ourselves on our growing maturity. Boundaries, properly practiced, protect us from anything short of a boundary violation.

If, however, we had been tossed back into an infantile ego state by a posttraumatic revisiting of an infant wound caused by a recent painful conversation, the first thing we must do is to parent ourselves. We may have to call a metaphorical time-out. We leave our apologies to others for later. In a quiet place, we must in effect do chair work on ourselves. We invite our abused child to image herself before us, and we tell her that we empathized with the emotion she was feeling, such as pain, fear, shame, or anger. We reassure her that we know how it was inflicted and how she adapted to fit that emotion into the family system. We tell her we feel her pain, but that she now has a functional adult to take care of her, an adult who will assuage her and keep her from harm. Of course, we are both the child and the adult.

This self-cleansing will help us reestablish our boundaries. When we react out of conditioning and we do not intellectually challenge our responses, we strengthen the conditioning. However, if we consistently challenge it, we weaken it and eventually remove it. As they say in the song, "Getting better all the time."

Ground Rules for Talking to Your Partner

1. *Don't accuse.* Accusing automatically puts you in the one-up position. It keeps you from communicating the data from which your feeling has sprung and disqualifies your partner from knowing why you are behaving the way you are.

2. *Don't tell your partner what he or she should be feeling.* This is instantly going to the one-up position. It is intensely demeaning to tell others that you know more about their emotional life than they themselves do. Most of us can't figure out why we are feeling the way we do, much less why others feel the way they do.

3. *Don't give advice.* Advising others is telling them how they should be solving their problems. You are telling them they have a problem without finding out from them if they believe they have a problem. In essence what you are doing is trying to take over their life. The reaction to that is they become defensive and shut you out.

4. *Don't judge.* So many of us sanctify the concept of "Wrong" as if it were the opposite of an absolute "Right," which we know, and others don't—but should. It is nothing so grand. For most people, "Wrong" means "when you operate outside my value system." We have beliefs about things such as how toilet paper should be put in the holder. Judgment interferes in the talking boundary when we say, "It's not appropriate to put the toilet paper in backwards," because we take a one-up position and wall ourselves off from our partner's response. The corrective for this behavior is to notice that you are about to do it and then refrain. Or if it does come out, to talk about how you came to your beliefs, such as, "In my family of origin

that's the way we used to put in the toilet paper. Isn't it interesting that we have different ideas."

5. *Don't guess at your partner's motivation.* You are saying that your thought processes are better than your partner's and that your partner doesn't even know what his or her own motivation is. You present yourself as an erudite person identifying the real reason behind the other's behavior and what the result is going to be. If you need to talk about motivation at all, do it in the form of "When I engage in that behavior, the reason I find myself doing it is. . . . "

6. *Don't be sarcastic.* Sarcasm is very brutal. The Greek etymological root of the word is *sarkasmos*, from *sarkazein*, to bite the lips in rage, from *sarx*, *sark-*, "flesh." Sarcasm is the basis of locker-room banter and seems to have infected all levels of American discourse. But for people who grew up in a sarcastic family, it is the form of humor they first learned. However, family members who are sarcastic to one another are not being relational; they are "biting the flesh." When children learn their humor from such a family, they use it as the family did—nonrelationally, with the intent to abuse from the one-up position. Sarcasm is a way of backing away from intimacy by disguising hostility or emotional embarrassment as humor.

7. *Don't use hard-to-understand private jargon.* Private jargon is harmful when it replaces an honest attempt to inform. It puts the user behind a wall of inscrutable superiority. It's a way of pushing the other person out of the conversation. It implies that you are being either contemptuous or manipulative through superiority.

8. *Don't say, "You really don't understand me."* This claim is tantamount to saying that any kind of a good relationship between you and your partner is impossible, because you have given up. It disqualifies your partner from the conversation and, therefore, from further attempts at intimacy. Often, however, it is a desperate way of inviting someone to keep trying to know you by dramatizing your pain. Then it is a cry for intimacy, even if it is a dysfunctional one.

9. *Don't call your partner names.* In-your-face name-calling is a boundary violation and an attack on another person's worth. If you have engaged in name-calling, it would be appropriate for the person you have abused to become angry with you, to wall off from attack, and from behind that wall to deny your humanity. In a less pernicious form, giving your partner your own private name is a way of owning the person that simplifies his or her complex humanity so that you can hold it in your fist. When you have a pet nickname for someone and only you can use it, you own that person in a way, and you are bottling up another person's humanity in the lifelessness of a label.

In the vignettes that follow, uses and abuses of the talking and listening boundaries assume familiar life.

Stuck at the Airport

Charles, an advertising account executive, and his attractive wife, Natalie, whom he has brought along to charm the client, have just arrived at the airport after having flown in from Europe.

Charles has forgotten to call his secretary to arrange for a driver to pick them up and now they will have to wait an hour and a half after an exhausting trip. He has just admitted that he has forgotten. Natalie talks to him this way:

"All you can think of is business (1. *Accusation*). If I were you, I would be ashamed of myself (2. *Telling him how to feel*). Why don't you use your Palm Pilot to help you remember so you wouldn't make blunders like this? (3. *Advice*). Your behavior is positively immoral (4. *Judgment*). Your only reason for taking me on this trip was to make up for all the time you neglect me (5. *Guessing at motivation*). I suppose that's what you 'Masters of the Universe' call business as usual (6. *Sarcasm*). If this isn't a case of passive-aggressive camouflage, I'll eat my hat. Well, *"Plus ça change, plus c'est la même chose* (7. *Private jargon*). But why am I telling this to you in the first place? (8. *'You really don't understand me'*). Let's face it, you are a self-centered jerk" (9. *Name-calling*)."

Fortunately for our didactic purposes, Natalie has broken all the ground rules for talking to one's partner. If she had used her talking boundary instead of violating each principle of functional talking, she might have said,

"As I am standing here, I am realizing that it is going to take an hour and a half for the driver to get here. I am feeling pretty angry about that. This has happened three times in the past year and it is a problem for me. Can we talk about this problem and try to resolve it?"

TV and the Roommates

Two roommates, Josh and Sam, live in a city in a small apartment. Josh watches television in the common den whenever he is home, which is a lot. This creates a burden on Sam's privacy, and he has become increasingly irritated. Sam has previously made low-key, painfully self-conscious requests that Josh cut back on the television usage, but he has never clearly told him how aggravating it is to him. Finally able to hold in his irritation no longer, Sam walks up to his roommate's TV lounger, stands two feet away from him, and, looming over him, says,

> "I've had all I can take of this. You are so disrespectful. We've lived together for six months now, and you continually have the TV on. You should be more aware of your obligations to me. You are really insensitive. Probably you're trying to show me who's boss here. Yeah, like you're Mr. Big Shot. Maybe there's just something wrong with your hearing. You are self-centered and egotistical, and you have no idea how to cooperate. You're interfering with my life, and I am not willing to do this anymore. Why do you have to act like such a putz?"

Compare the above with a boundaried talking approach. After approaching Josh and standing or sitting at a nonthreatening distance from him, Sam says something like this,

> "Can we talk about something that's been bothering me? I know that you like to watch TV and the level that you do it at is not comfortable for me. And what I think is that you do not care about my comfort and I feel

some shame and anger. Can we negotiate the times that you watch or that sometimes you will watch it using a headset if I got one for you? Would it be all right with you if I come in and ask you to turn it down when it is too loud?"

As in life, this first attempt at boundaried talking may not have the desired effect. What follows is an inappropriate response on the part of the television addict.

"Thanks a lot, Rabbit Ears. Yes, I knew that there was something wrong with you. You look like you've had your head up your ass for the past ten days. It's about time that you finally said what's on your mind. You know I've noticed that you usually can't speak about what's on your mind, and that really annoys me. Why do you have to be such a wimp? As far as the television goes, considering the rent I pay, I have a right to watch television whenever I want to, and if you don't like it, there is a public library you can go to. It's just down the block."

Let us imagine that Sam has a black belt in listening boundaries and has managed to keep his cool (maybe he has even said the "Serenity Prayer"). He responds,

"I know that bringing up things that bother me is one of my failings. It is pretty uncomfortable for me. It took me a long time for me to get up enough nerve to talk to you about this, and this may be something we just can't get past. We may have to decide that we can't be roommates. But I am willing to talk about it and see if we can find some middle ground."

Sam does not address the abusive names he was called. Here, he diplomatically uses a wall of protection, as there is no truth in the names that matches his sense of himself. He has a right to cut off for the sake of the relationship if he still has a stake in keeping it going.

Too Much Time and Money Spent in a Bar

Dave and Emily are newly married and are very much in love. At the end of the month, when Emily is balancing the checkbook, she notices that Dave is spending a lot of money at a bar. She doesn't think he is an alcoholic; maybe she doesn't even know what an alcoholic is, but she is very upset about all the money he is spending. She is frightened to speak to him, because she doesn't want to annoy him, but finally it becomes too much for her and, using her talking boundary, she says the following to him,

> "I have been going through the checkbook, and I have found out that you have been spending money at a local bar. Our finances are pretty stretched as it is, and I am angry that you spend all this money without talking to me about it. And I have all sorts of suspicions about what you are doing down at the bar—about women who might be there and about why I am being left out of your social life, and I am really angry about this."

Dave's toxic, dysfunctional response is

"Look, Em, did you ever hear of the expression, 'All work and no play'? I've got to let my hair down sometimes, and as far as this woman stuff goes, don't you trust me at all? You are really being a meddler. I guess you can't help being just like your mother, seeing an infidelity around every corner. How old is that news? How can I make myself clear to you? Don't you understand my needs at all? I mean, how long have we been married? I don't see that you have a right to be so damn suspicious. Be my wife—not some kind of private eye."

Here is what he could have said if he were exercising his talking and listening boundaries properly:

"First of all, Em, I am really sorry that you feel the way you do. If I had seen all those checks cashed at the bar, I might have wondered what was going on also. But you know how much stress I have been under at work, and I admit that at the end of the day, I have been going to the bar to have a few vodkas and shoot the breeze with the rest of the guys. A few times, instead of going to the bank, I cashed a check at the bar. As for a woman, that is not true, I promise. As for keeping you out of my social life, you know I never thought of that aspect of it when I was at the bar. I guess it has been selfish of me not to have seen it that way. I owe you an apology for that and for the money.

"Can we do this? What I suggest is that we sit down and go over our finances and set up some kind of a bud-

get. And then we can establish how much disposable income we have after putting aside for the basics, so that
we can each have an equal amount of money to do with
what we want each month. If one of us wants to spend
more money than that, we talk about it and negotiate
something reasonable and fair."

Maybe that will not be the end of their discussion. Maybe
there is an issue concerning Dave's reliance on alcohol in order
to relax. Perhaps Emily has an abandonment issue going back to
her mother's jealousy problems with her own husband. By behaving civilly to one another, by exercising their talking and listening boundaries, they are caring for their intimacy. They are
keeping themselves open to one another, and when the time
comes for them to discuss other issues, they will have developed
skill in and commitment to the healthy practice of boundaries.

The Phone Bill

Loretta, examining her monthly phone bill, notices that there
are phone charges for calls to Europe that she didn't make. Because of the dates involved, she assumes the calls were made by
Sophia, an Italian friend of hers who had been staying at her
home during this time period. Wanting to find out more about
the phone charges, she calls Sophia, who is now back in Italy,
and says,

"Sophia, I just found some phone charges to Rome
made from my phone when you were staying here. I
know that you must have made them and I am angry

that you essentially stole from me by using my phone without permission. Since when have you become so sneaky? I guess you just don't trust me enough to tell me the truth. What have I done to deserve such treatment? I thought you knew better. What do you have to say for yourself?"

The above response is very unboundaried. It is accusatory; it guesses at motives. It is sarcastic and leaves no room for negotiation.

If Loretta had exercised proper talking boundaries, she would have been able to focus on telling the truth, but telling the truth respectfully. It might sound like this:

"I found phone charges for calls to Italy on my bill during the time you were visiting me. I don't think I made these phone calls and I am wondering if you made them."

In this way she opens up a conversation without accusing, so that she can gather data before making any statement that in fairness requires them. If Sophia were to respond functionally, she might say,

"Yes, I did make those phone calls and I forgot to tell you about them. I apologize for that. Tell me what I owe you and I will mail it to you today."

In this scenario, the listener, Sophia, admits the truth of what has been told her. She does not have to make excuses. She declares herself ready to make amends, and the matter is at a close. Perhaps Loretta may wonder at how her friend managed to forget to pay for these calls, but this would be a good time to be diplomatic for the relationship and let it pass, content that the bill will be paid and that Sophia has made an honest statement of her part in the affair.

If, on the other hand, Sophia decided to get on her high horse and indulge a dysfunctional attitude, she might say something like this:

"Well, so that is your notion of being a hostess, is it? You are going to charge me as if I were a paying customer! That is not my idea of hospitality. What are you, an innkeeper? I can assure you that if you came to my home, you could use the phone all you wanted. "*Mi casa es su casa.*" Well, if you are going to be a skinflint, I might as well throw in an additional interest charge. Next time I'll stay at a hotel."

Still not content with the poison she has been spreading, Sophia reaches a crescendo, adding,

"Now, I want you to understand something—I love you. You must know that if you know anything at all. And I certainly did not expect this kind of payback. I guess I will never understand you."

It will take practiced use of the listening boundary to respond functionally to such hostile and manipulative communication. The weapon of telling the person you are attacking that you "love" them is an especially septic tactic. Abusive parents specialize in it. Here is the way Loretta's healthy response might sound:

"As I listen to you, I realize that you have just called me unloving and accused me of being ungenerous and in-hospitable. What I think is going on here is that you and I work out of two different value systems about how to have someone in their home. And about that I am feel-ing some sadness, because I can see that it has really af-fected our relationship.

"Listen, though, what I would like you to know is that in the future, when you are staying here—and you are perfectly welcome to stay with me—when you use my phone for international calls, I would like you to tell me that you have done so. And, if the total amount is, let's say, over twenty dollars, I would like you to pay me back.

"Perhaps, we can talk about this at a later date when both of us are not so upset. Would you be willing to do that?"

In the course of her unboundaried response, Sophia, in ad-dition to other boundary failures, has committed a boundary vi-olation—she called her friend a name and directly attacked her worth. Therefore, Loretta's boundaried response to her might involve something that acknowledges the boundary violation:

"When you called me unloving, inhospitable, and a skinflint, what I believe about this is that you were call-ing me names and that you were being abusive to me, attacking my value as a human being, and about that I am very angry. In the future, when we have discussions over things that we disagree about, I would really appre-ciate it if you didn't call me names."

The Film Director's Breakfast

Nick, a film director, was always scouting out exotic locations for the movie company or tied up with the shoot, while his wife, Monica, was home with the children. Nick was a demon worker, and he made the people who worked for him toe the line. Monica felt she was being crushed and that Nick was deaf to her predicament or what she needed from him. The friction between husband and wife had reached incendiary levels. They were in my couples boundary workshop to learn how to use boundaries with one another.

I had asked them the night before to go back to their hotel and write out some things that had happened between the two of them that distressed them but that they had never shared with one another before.

Nick went first. I had seen in his written report that he felt his wife was not feeding the children properly. He thought that she was feeding the children too much junk food, too much chocolate-flavored cereal at breakfast. He was a health-food devotee. He wanted the four-year-old to eat muesli. He was highly distressed about his wife's behavior.

Nick burst out at Monica obnoxiously, talking without any functional boundaries:

"What you do is feed the children this hideous junk food, and what I think about that is that you are a terrible mother, and I am so angry about that that I want to divorce you."

Nick went into an all-out attack on his wife over the cereal. I told him that he needed to stop talking. I told him that he was being offensive and using spurious words to describe what his wife did. I told him that he was not at all diplomatic and that I wanted him to think about how he could say the same thing to his wife without being as obnoxious as he was being. And that is when he sat there and sat there and sat there and couldn't think of what to say. Nick was incapable of reaching into the chaos of his emotions to say what was on his mind without being choked by self-righteous anger.

I suggested to him this:

"Monica, what I noticed was that you have been feeding the children Chocolate Puffs, and what I think is that it doesn't have enough nourishment in it. As I think about your feeding them this nonnutritional cereal, I feel a lot of anger. I would like to talk about what you are feeding them, because I have some other ideas about what might be better for them."

After hearing me out, Nick burst out again, "But I don't want her feeding the children junk food at all."

I pointed out to him that he wanted his wife to feed the kids muesli, which was filled with hard-to-digest fiber and which probably didn't taste good to a young child. I suggested to him that he probably wanted to negotiate a deal with his wife whereby she could feed the kids a cereal that might not be the cereal that he wanted them to eat, but that wouldn't be the chocolate-flavored, nonnutritional stuff he detested.

Monica informed us that the chocolate-flavored puffs actually were nutritionally sound and that they had been made with whole grains. The result was that they decided on a third cereal that had more fiber than what she had been feeding the kids but less nourishment than what he wanted.

What I confronted Nick about was how he operated in the extremes, that he was completely immoderate, and that for him anything but what he could find in a health-food store was junk. For her part, Monica admitted that she did sometimes feed the kids food that was less nutritional than desired and sweeter than recommended just to keep them quiet.

They were literally going to get divorced over this issue. The Chocolate Puffs were about to cause the director to lose half of his several millions. Nick's problem was that he couldn't think of how to talk to Monica respectfully and then went rigid about what the solution had to be. So Nick had to work on speaking respectfully and learning how to negotiate without getting everything he wanted. He had to give up talking to her from a one-up position and becoming toxic and abusive simply because he felt he was right.

When Monica heard his attacks, she handled it quite well. She told me that she had gone to a wall, where she stopped listening to him when he used the demeaning words to her.

Monica did well in negotiating. She was willing to go to a third cereal that would be harder to get the children to eat; she did so in the interests of the relationship.

Time Difference

An overworked and phenomenally successful international sales director of a computer company and his wife come to my workshop. Ronald's charismatic power struck me immediately. Charismatic people want to capture you and hold you hostage to their

will. His complaint was that his wife, Charlotte, hadn't acknowledged his latest birthday. He was experiencing a lot of shame
and pain about it, but he couldn't reveal that information to me.
He was as blocked as if his mouth had been sewn shut.

What Charlotte later reported was that he had been on a
business trip and was eight time zones ahead of where she was.
She had remembered his birthday, but didn't want to awaken
him in the middle of the night. By the time it was a good hour to
call, Charlotte was at the art gallery she ran in the city, had become distracted, and plain forgot. It wasn't because she didn't
love him. She just forgot.

Charlotte shared these facts with Ronald and spoke of her
feelings for him: he was a wonderful person and she loved him
deeply. Then she apologized for forgetting and told him that she
could understand how distressed he had become. She was concerned about his distress. She avoided getting into defending
herself by saying that he was eight time zones ahead and that he
should have understood that. She used her talking boundary
quite well.

But although Charlotte was capable of talking relationally
about his distress, Ronald remained tied in agonizing knots
about the pain of not having his birthday acknowledged. If I
hadn't learned from Charlotte the details of why she hadn't
called him and what his reaction had been, he on his own would
never have told me about his pain.

It was only when I examined Ronald's trauma issues that we
made some progress. Ronald had a mother who was neglectful
and abandoned him when he was five years old. The childhood
beliefs he developed because of his mother's behavior were that
he was worthless and that any woman he let get close would
abandon him. That is why he couldn't speak up. He was in a

very young ego state (younger than five), became dissociated, and couldn't talk. In this instance an issue from his family of origin had been triggered.

At that point, I moved with Ronald into chair work with his mother. We imaged her into the room and talked with her about abandoning him at age five and what he thought about himself, which was that he was a worthless, defective kid. He released a lot of the child pain and shame connected with that issue.

Then I had Ronald talk to his mother from an adult perspective and tell her what he thought about her leaving him like that: that it was irresponsible as a parent and he was very sad that she never reconnected with him. I helped him to understand that his childhood feeling of worthlessness was about her being an inadequate parent and not about his being worthless. Ronald had been carrying around that shame all his adult life. Finally he was able to give it back to his mother—where it belonged. Happy Birthday!

Ground Rules for Exercising the Internal Listening Boundary

1. Set your external physical boundary in order to be more comfortable as you listen.

2. Remind yourself not to take the blame.

3. Remind yourself the emotions you experience as you listen have to be regulated by breath work so that they do not become too powerful and radiate toxically into the air.

4. Remind yourself that you are listening to find out who the other person is, not to formulate your defense.

5. Review that you protect yourself as you listen by determining if what is being said is "true," "not true," or "questionable."

6. If what you are hearing is "true," allow yourself to feel emotions about this truth.

7. If what you are hearing is "not true," detach from feeling emotions about what is being said.

8. If what you are hearing is "questionable," when the person is finished talking, ask for the data you need in order to decide if it is "true" or "not true." Ask for the data in four sentences or less without complaining, blaming, or explaining why you need the data. This will help the other person listen.

9. If negotiation is necessary, start the process.

You use your listening boundary when others start talking to you. They are sharing what they have observed, what they heard and smelled, and so forth, what they thought and felt about it, and what they want to do about it.

They are projecting ideas and emotions toward you. The listening boundary receives that information and energy and processes it in a way that requires you to be vulnerable enough to be receptive (open), but not so vulnerable that you can be damaged by untruth. Being too vulnerable is a boundary failure. Being invulnerable means that you put up a wall and are not able to listen.

The first thing you should do when someone starts talking to you about a subject that calls up negative energy is to set the external physical boundary, so you can be comfortable while you listen. You may want to stand back a little bit or walk around the other side of a counter. You might pick up a binder and hold it to your chest. If you need some time to set the distance that will make you comfortable, ask the person to hold it for a minute.

Then you have to set your internal listening boundary before you can functionally listen. If someone catches you off guard with an unexpectedly quick-talking approach, ask them to stop for a while until you can get your internal listening boundary prepared.

As the person starts talking, remind yourself not to take the blame, which means that you are not responsible for how this person assessed what happened. You are not responsible for how she says things, hears things, or smells things. You didn't make her think anything. You didn't make her feel anything or do anything. She is responsible for those things.

The third thing you must do is to regulate the emotions you feel as you listen, so that they remain moderate and do not radiate out into the air and become toxic.

The fourth thing you do is remind yourself that you are listening to find out who the speaker is, not to formulate your defense. This is important. You want to assume the posture of a detective going on an investigation, discovering this person's thoughts, deeds, and feelings. Many people forget that they are listening to find out who the person is who is speaking to them. Instead, they go to a wall of talking inside their heads, concentrating all the while on how the person they are listening to is wrong. As a result they hear nothing but their own static.

In Rule 4, what you are essentially doing is opening yourself up to intimacy, while moderating your vulnerability. In Rule 5 you begin to protect yourself by determining if the sensory input of what the person saw or heard and what he or she made up about it is for you true, untrue, or questionable.

What happens between Rules 4 and 5 is that you step into the center between no boundaries and a wall. In this place in the center you listen with the attitude that you are discovering who the speaker is. You are not going to take in the untrue stuff—only what for you is true, and you allow yourself to have feelings only about those true things.

If you decide that what you are hearing is not true, you detach from your feeling about it or let your feelings pass through you without effect—like a ghost. You acknowledge that the speaker has a right to be different. You stay respectful of his or her right to be different, but you do not let it bash you around. You don't let something that is not true bash you around. You get attached to or have emotions about only what you know is a truth that matches your truth—and that is where vulnerability is.

Sometimes when we have to listen to some truth about ourselves that is negative, we have unpleasant emotions and are vulnerable to the unpleasant truth. Even measured vulnerability is vulnerability, and vulnerability is often painful. That is life. It comes with being intimate. It is the same with the talking boundary. Even with the talking boundary in place, you are being vulnerable, because you are giving people information about yourself that they could use against you or about which they may have ideas, thoughts, and emotions that may cause them to distance themselves from you and cause you pain. So both revealing yourself and letting in unpleasant truth make you vulnerable. However, without vulnerability there is no love.

If what the speaker tells you about the sensory input is questionable, when the speaker is finished talking, share that you are not sure what is being talked about and ask for more data. As you get additional sensory input, see if you can change the questionable data into something that is either true or untrue for you.

If the data remains questionable or becomes untrue, back off and don't have feelings about it until it becomes a truth. If it remains questionable, ask the person to continue giving you data. If you decide that with even more data it still remains untrue, back off, notice how it differs from your truth, and remain respectful.

At this impasse, in order to keep the intimacy process working, you would move to your talking boundary and share with the person who has not made matters clear to you how your listening boundary actually operated in terms of true, untrue, and questionable. Diplomatically, you would always lead with what you agree with. "Hey, listen, when you talked about this and that and had those thoughts and feelings, I have to share with you that I thought the very same thing."

Since you have already shared about what was questionable, the next thing you could share is what was not true for you. Here you have to think *diplomatically.* You have to assess if this person is in a frame of mind or has enough energy to listen to what you disagree with. If you think the person is in an unreceptive state, you might share that. You offer to hold off until the person is more receptive.

If you are in agreement that what is being said constitutes a problem for you both, you share that you see it as a problem and that you would like to talk more about the problem and move on to some sort of a negotiation. Like partners, you work out a deal and then go out into the world and do what you agreed to do.

Resentment is one of the most common causes of listening boundary failure. We experience resentment when we believe that somebody has treated us disrespectfully and damaged our self-esteem. Often, though, in reaction to something someone has told us, we experience a very uncomfortable emotion and go to resentment or self-pity, even though there has been no boundary violation. Our boundaries have been violated only if someone has yelled or screamed, called us names, lied to us, or tried to control or manipulate us. In the absence of these provocations, the resentment is invariably provoked by some false information that we have made up in our own heads as to the meaning of what has been said to us. And, invariably, we make up such information because we are feeling bad about ourselves before the provocation. We make ourselves the victims of a violation that did not occur, and for that reason I call resentment "victim anger." When we go to a state of self-pity, I call that "victim pain."

The Angry Secretary

Eileen is the managing editor of a small publishing firm; she also goes out with its editor-in-chief. One morning Eileen told Julian, her boss-boyfriend, to be careful of the secretary "because she was in a foul mood." Julian became furious with Eileen over this remark. The background of Julian's emotionality is that his company is in bad financial condition and he has been blaming himself for a lot of the problems. When Eileen reported the secretary's emotional state, Julian flushed with anger that his attention was being drawn to such a relatively unimportant issue. He hotly scolded Eileen that he had so much more on his mind than that "goddamned secretary." In the secrecy of his own self-pity (victim pain) he thought, "If my girlfriend is going to show sympathy for anyone, why shouldn't it be for me?"

In order to feed his resentment, Julian made up the idea that his girlfriend cared more about the secretary and her mood than she cared about how much stress he was under. When Julian made that up about Eileen, he made up that his girlfriend didn't love him. Buried under all of this was the belief that he was being victimized by his girlfriend.

In reality Eileen was giving him information that he could use to steer clear of the secretary or giving him warning to prepare an appropriate defense so that his day would not be more troublesome than it already was.

The Profligate Son

Dorothy's listening boundary was challenged when Jack, her young, married son, accused her of not loving him because she had stopped giving him a weekly supplement to his earnings. Jack, who is a recovering alcoholic, and his wife have an infant. Because the wife chose to stay at home until the child was a little older, she could not bring earnings into the household. Dorothy understood and sympathized with the problem and agreed to supplement her son's income for a while, as long as he was sober, going to AA meetings, and working every day. After a period of abstinence and steady work, Jack resumed his drinking and dope smoking and started missing days at work. He asked for more money to make up for his missed work.

When Dorothy realized what was going on, she believed that by continuing to give Jack added money she was enabling him in his habit and in his denial. Finally she decided to limit the amount of money she was willing to give and told him that if he drank again or did not work steadily, she would stop giving him money. He continued to slip and slide. Finally, the day came when Dorothy chose to invoke the penalty for Jack's having broken their agreement.

She told her son that she felt some fear and anger about his substance abuse and his not working steadily. He responded by saying that her withholding of money meant that she did not love or care about him. He said that, as his mother, she owed him the money anyway. He said that he was angry.

Dorothy told Jack that she did not want to enable him. She told him that she loved him and that was why the rules surrounding money and how he must behave in order to keep receiving it would remain in place. The accusations that she did not love her son or care for him hurt, but because they were not true, she allowed them to pass through her, and she breathed into the pain so that it did not infect the room. Jack left angrily with his own emotions intact, but with no carried dysfunctional energy from his mother as an additional burden to him. There was no immediate resolution.

Sure, it was tough love, but Dorothy's healthy listening boundary kept her from joining in Jack's dysfunctional self-pity. Most important, the door remained open for him to continue to receive support if he kept his side of the bargain. She told her truth without withholding her love. The ball was now squarely in his court, the court from which he had manipulatively tried to move it by accusing his mother of not loving him and by saying that the money was owed him regardless of his behavior. And although that was painful for Dorothy, there was no healthy alternative.

At a time like this, when doing the right thing is so painful, people who permit themselves to pray should consider themselves fortunate.

God, grant me the serenity
to accept the things I cannot change;
the courage to change the things I can;
and the wisdom to know the difference.

Paying for Half the Dinner Check

When I was a young nurse working at the Meadows, I had begun to date Pat Mellody, the director of the Meadows, who was to become my husband. In those days I was a pretty mixed-up person, as readers have already learned from Chapter 1. Because I had such a weak hold on my self-esteem, I often insisted on grandly faking it. One such attempt was at the dinners that Pat and I had when we were dating. No matter that my nurse's salary was pretty meager, I would insist that I pick up my half of the check. I would have it no other way, and I was adamant, making it a matter of principle. Finally, after one more scene of my insisting that I pay half, Pat said,

> "Pia, your insistence on picking up half the check is hampering our relationship, because I have much more money than you do. I am becoming reluctant to ask you out to dinner, even though I want to, because I don't want to hurt you financially. I'd like to suggest to you that we negotiate, so that when half the check is more than what you and I identify as a comfortable amount for you, you allow me to pick up the rest."

I was very relieved and actually got positive feelings about my self-worth as a result of this mature handling of the reality issue. Notice that Pat did not commit the talking boundary violation of guessing at my motives by saying some such thing as "I know that you are trying to be a big shot by covering up your basic insecurity." Nor did he call me names, as in "Why don't you stop being such a silly little thing?" Nor was he snide or sarcastic by saying, "Hell, I know how much money you make. After all, I pay your salary. Pia, get real!" Instead, Pat treated me like an adult, and I responded like one.

You Didn't Come to My Lecture

It is tempting to avoid our accountability for having erred in a relationship when we can hide behind something of which we are innocent—using the innocent part to divert attention from the guilty part. Suppose Ned says to me that last Wednesday night I promised to attend a lecture that he was giving on Apache painting but that I didn't show up. He tells me that the idea he makes up about this is that I don't love or care for him, and he says that he feels some anger and pain.

True? Untrue? Questionable? I did go to the lecture, but there were so many people clustered around Ned at the conclusion of it, I couldn't get close enough, and after waiting twenty minutes, because I had things to do at home, I left. Afterwards, I thought about calling him to say that I had been there, but I got busy and forgot.

If I were listening to Ned's description of what I did and what he made up about it with my listening boundary operating dysfunctionally, I would tell him that if he had only been more attentive, he would have seen me there, and that if he had cared about me a little more, he wouldn't have allowed himself to be distracted by the crowd that surrounded him at the end of his lecture. If I had talked so dysfunctionally, I also would probably have guessed at his motives in order to hide my own guilt at being late, leaving early, and forgetting to call him later on. I might have said with some sarcasm, "Clearly you enjoy being the center of attention, even if it means ignoring your good friends."

However, if I were to respond with my listening boundary operating correctly, I would tell Ned that I did go to the lecture, but when I saw the crowds around him, I left. I would admit that not calling him afterwards was my failure and that I would like to apologize for that. I would say that I wanted to share with him that I really did care for him.

The Artist and the Critic

When you have produced a work you think is beautiful and meaningful, and a critic comes up to you and says she thinks it is terrible, if you are using your listening boundary correctly, you compare what that critic thinks against what you think. Is what she is saying true or false or questionable according to what you think? If you think that the work is beautiful, what you do is notice that you and the critic have two different ideas, and you value and feel good about your own. You find it interesting that she has an opinion different from yours. This is respectful detachment. You don't demean or attack her or take in an idea from her that doesn't fit your truth.

You could also, after listening carefully about what she has said about your work, decide to change your mind because what she has said changes the truth of what you originally thought. "Let me think about this." You may decide that some of her ideas are actually true. You then take the critic's information in as a truth and adjust your own feeling about it. When you do that, your boundary has worked as a filter. It gives you a chance to think about what the critic was saying. In the first scenario you rejected what she was saying, but recognized that she had a right to her viewpoint. In the second scenario, you changed your own mind about your own product, and you took it in and may have had some pain and embarrassment before acknowledging the truth of what you learned. That pain is part of life, especially the creative life. *"C'est la vie!"*

Parent or Critic?

On the weekend before the opening of her movie, Leila, the young screenwriter and director, had been invited to appear on a network television program to talk about her upcoming film. During the interview Leila did no commercial hyping of her film. Instead, the young filmmaker talked about the very human confusion and uncertainties that went into the creation of the film. In talking about the unpredictability of the creative process, Leila's appearance was a candid picture of the artist's vulnerability.

Vanessa, Leila's mother, who has seen private screenings of the new film, admires it and is proud of her daughter's imagination and professionalism, and she has told Leila so. This kind of open communication between them is relatively new, because Vanessa, the divorced mother, drank alcoholically for most of Leila's formative years and was abusive and authoritarian. Now that Vanessa is sober and in recovery, she regrets the pain she has caused her family, in particular Leila, and welcomes the opportunity to share her approval of Leila's television interview.

Vanessa called Leila and told her that the interview was wonderful and fascinating. She said that it was unusually refreshing for Leila not to hype the movie with commercial motives foremost. Vanessa told Leila that to speak of the befuddlements of the creative process was honest and interesting. The mother then said, "But I've got to be honest with you, people will wonder why you didn't take the opportunity to hype the film the way they usually do in Hollywood." Vanessa sensed some distress in her daughter's voice when Leila, after thanking her for the nice things her mother said, said that the producers of the film don't feel that the interview missed a commercial opportunity. "In fact," Leila said, "they think that it will bring a lot of attention to the film and sell tickets."

Later in the day, Leila called her mother back, heralding what she had to say by admitting how upset she was with her mother's criticism. She said that she was hurt and angry that her mother would criticize her at such an inopportune moment. Leila said, "At this point I need a mother, not a critic." Vanessa felt pain and anger. She had a shame attack.

Vanessa told her daughter that she meant to compliment her and to express her admiration for Leila's talking about the creative act and not about ticket sales. Vanessa said it pained her and shamed her to hear how she hurt her daughter. She said it was not her intention to do that. She told Leila that she was really upset. The daughter listened politely, but it was clear that the deeply distressing emotions Leila felt had deep roots. Mother and daughter terminated their conversation politely, but both were shook up.

During their second phone call, Vanessa shared with Leila that she blamed herself for having hurt her. In that act, the mother was inappropriately taking responsibility for the pain the daughter felt as a result of what Leila herself *made up* about what Vanessa said. And that was a *boundary failure* of the mother's. Vanessa was taking blame for what her daughter had made up and felt about Vanessa's words. At this point, if the scene could be reenacted, it would be important for Vanessa to go to her talking boundary and say,

> "From what you have just said to me about my comments that your television interview was not commercial, I think that you saw them as critical as opposed to supportive. I thought that what I was saying was supporting

you and that I felt proud of the stance you took. Rather than brag about the movie, you actually talked about the nature of the creative act. I am noticing that we have some real different ideas about the intent of what I said. About that I am feeling some shame."

Vanessa also felt some anger, but *diplomatically for the relationship* that would not have been appropriate to share at that time, as Leila was not ready to hear it. Vanessa would just say that she felt a great deal of shame or embarrassment about being thought of as a person who would painfully criticize her daughter on the occasion of such an important event in her daughter's life.

The mother would then listen to what the daughter had to say to her. If the daughter hung on to her idea of what the mother meant as opposed to the mother's idea of what she meant, the mother would have to respect that her daughter has a different idea about what the mother said and that she has a right to have it. The daughter's belief reflects her history with the alcoholic mother when in her drunken past she was critical of her with tormenting regularity.

In the face of her belief Vanessa could say to Leila something like

"I know what happened between the two of us when you were a child and I was a young mother. I know that what came out of my mouth was because I was drunk and I didn't know how to parent anyway. I know that I was quite critical and abusive, and I can see that you would believe that I was criticizing you now because that's the way it always was. And what I would like to say to you is that I apologize for all the times I was so inappropriate and abusive to you as a child. I would like to share with you that I am really proud of what you have done."

One can never know what the results of such appropriate candor will be, but if we are to stand a chance at healthy relationality, we have to put in the effort. It will do us no good to be disabled by our remorse at our past transgressions. It is our job in relationships to put in the work and let go of the results. We do not blame ourselves for what others are feeling, even though we know our part in past abuses. In AA they say, "We row, God steers."

Our Marriage Is No Longer Exciting

Clive felt that his once exciting marriage had become dull and unstimulating. He felt that it was his wife's fault. He was so upset that he decided to confront Virginia with his feelings. Clive said,

"I don't recognize you these days as being the same woman I married. We used to share so many interests: the same books, the theater, we used to travel to places, your friends were interesting to me, and my friends seemed to interest you. We used to look forward to sex. What has happened to your intellectual curiosity? Why is it that you are content sitting in front of that stupid television watching daytime soap operas? I can't go on living like this. You know we don't live forever, and I am forty-seven years old now. I work hard enough at my job, and you sit here at home and do nothing but wonder what diet you should be on. I am fed up with it, and unless you see the light, I don't see that there is any hope for this marriage."

Clearly Clive was accusatory and demeaning. He assumed that his observations were the only relevant data and appeared to offer no hope or reasonable expectation of a working solution to their problems. What might Clive have said if he had exercised a healthy talking boundary? It might have sounded something like this:

"Recently I have been concerned because life doesn't seem to have a lot of interest for me, especially in my relationship with you. It used to be that we had a lot of fun together and did things together, but it seems we have grown apart for some reason and I don't know what that is. I don't know whether my interests have changed or your interests have changed, but we don't seem to be on the same path anymore. I cherish my memories of what it was like being with you, and I would like to try to regain some of that. I would like to have a dialogue with you to see if we can get some spark back in our marriage."

Virginia's response, either to the first dysfunctional remarks or to the second functional ones of her husband, damaged her listening boundary, and she struck back dysfunctionally:

"I don't know how you can attack me like this. I thought you loved me. I guess you've been lying to me all this time. You know we're not young anymore, so it's about time you grew up. I have responsibilities now. I have to take care of this household. Sure, you'd like to go off gallivanting around the rest of the world. Isn't that what your friend Jim did when he broke up with Marsha after eighteen years of marriage? Isn't it about time you recognized that it takes two to share? It's not always going to be your way. It's been forever since you've spoken honestly and intimately with me. What is this—male menopause? Did you ever stop to think how boring and self-absorbed you've become? Why don't you look in the mirror for a change? Why is it always the woman's fault?"

Is it possible to listen to such an indictment and remain centered enough to turn a potential emotional disaster into an occasion for a fresh start and productive sharing? A lot of people might respond by saying something like "Screw you and the horse you rode in on." But there is a better way, and it causes a lot less pain and produces a lot more good. A functional response to Virginia and the ensuing dialog might sound like this:

Clive: "I, too, have noticed that we don't seem to do things together, and that I have my circle of friends, you have your circle of friends, and that we are growing apart.

"I don't think that that is all bad. I don't think it is improper for you to have your interests and for me to have mine. But I would like to work with you so that we are doing more things together, and even have 'date night,' a time when we establish that we do things together. Let's talk about what you like to do and see if I can join you in good spirit, still leaving the way open for us to do things on our own when we want to."

Virginia: "What you have just said to me sounds fine, but I'm really scared. What are you feeling? Are you scared? I'm really nervous about this."

Clive: "Well, I'm nervous about this, too, and I have been for a long time. We've had so much together, and we've created so much together. I hate to lose it, but we do seem to be growing apart."

Virginia: "Do you think there's any hope for us?"

Clive: "I think it would be good if we found a third person to speak with, so that we could do some therapy together."

Virginia: "Do you really mean that?"

Clive: "Absolutely."

Virginia: "And would you mind if I gave you a hug?"

It is hard work—even revolutionary—to master the art of talking and listening boundaries. Our attempts to talk and listen to the people with whom we would like to be intimate are characteristically interrupted by signals sent to us from our traumatic past. They tell us that we need to defend ourselves, because if we don't, people will find out about our inadequacies and we will be embarrassed and humiliated. Most people who consider themselves "normal" live in this anxious condition and see nothing abnormal in the defensive or aggressive precautions they take to remain invulnerable.

Long ago, when I first heard recovering alcoholics at AA meetings describe themselves as "*grateful* recovering alcoholics," I wondered why they would be grateful for the suffering and pain their alcoholism had caused. Later on I came to see that it was only because their alcoholism had made them so desperate that they had been forced to learn about a better way of living and loving. Had these grateful recovering alcoholics been more "normal," they would never have found it necessary to learn that the status quo was an unhealthy place.

Most of us who have problems with relationships maintain our dysfunctional "normality" by viewing incoming emotion and thought as hostile and respond either by going silent (walled in) or turning aggressive (uncontained). In either case we seek to become invulnerable, and in becoming invulnerable we step outside of relationship and make intimacy impossible.

Our attempts to wall ourselves off from the remnants of childhood shame, fear, loneliness, and guilt generate our maladaptive "adult" personality. Still controlled by emotional forces that originate in our unexamined past, we view the truth about ourselves and the truth about others as potentially destructive to our inherent worth. We fear that the truth will reveal us for the defective people we are. We continue to be manipulated by strings that stretch back to our childhoods, unconsciously acting out the roles assigned to us by our dysfunctional caregivers.

While listening to Ronald, the international director of computer sales in "Time Difference" (p. 97), I realized that he was in the grips of a trauma so restrictive to him that he would be incapable of understanding his totally immoderate reaction to his wife's not having called him on his birthday. He was too unconscious of his traumatic past to exercise talking and listening boundaries and to be relational with his wife. With that realization, I decided to do trauma work with him and, along with it, that part of trauma work called chair work. For him it was necessary to learn the truth of his childhood; for without this truth, he was incapable of resisting the compulsive desire to attack and blame that destroyed his boundaries.

Without boundaries, there is no relationship. Without relationship there is no intimacy. Without intimacy there is no love, and without love the spiritual path is hidden from us.

Boundaries create the experience of truth and respect in which love can grow. We recognize that our inherent worth cannot be taken away from us by the display of our authentic selves. We are human and only that. We are born with inherent worth and it coexists with all our human flaws. Trauma work aims at identifying the abuse that first made us allergic to ourselves—to our flawed and imperfect humanity.

In the vignettes in the next chapter, the couples who have come for treatment need to be freed from posttraumatic stress before they can learn the practice of boundaries. All of them will go through the experience of chair work, which I describe in detail in the Appendix, "Feeling Reduction Workshop."

9

TRAUMA WORK

Precursor to Healthy Boundaries

"If you're hysterical, it's historical."
—AA maxim

SEXUAL TRAUMA

"He Makes Me Feel Dirty"

Trish was in her early thirties. She had been married to Benjamin for five years, and the marriage was in trouble. Benjamin complained that Trish was sexually cold and that she rejected his amorous advances. It hadn't always been that way, he said. When they were first married, they still went out drinking a lot, and, with alcohol allaying any lurking anxieties, their sex had been satisfactory, even though, as they would come to understand, not *intimate*.

Benjamin had in the past two years become so frustrated and insulted by Trish's developing sexual retreat that he had pretty much stopped approaching her. When he was frank with her about his sexual desires, she clammed up. When he went slow and courted her, she made believe she didn't notice. He was fed up with being treated as if something were wrong with him. He wanted and needed sex, and he did not want to look outside the marriage for it.

Trish reported that Benjamin would "leer" at her. His sexual approaches made her feel uneasy. The word she used was "slimy." Even as she said it, she turned red with embarrassment. She wondered how she could be saying such a thing about her husband, but even after owning up to the feeling, she didn't allow the psychological implications to sink in. She walled herself off from further examination of her emotional reaction to him. Instead, she reported in an irritated and self-justifying manner that, "All he thinks about is sex," and, "If he has a problem, he doesn't have to take it out on me. All he ever does is criticize me."

In therapy, Trish admitted that she had retreated from Benjamin and had made herself become sexually nonresponsive. But she "wasn't going to be abused." She could even read his mind. She said, "I know that he thinks of me as a sex object. That's why I feel so dirty when he gives me those looks." Trish was certain that there was nothing wrong with her sexually. It was just the way Benjamin went about things. It was all getting to be too much for her. "What has happened to our marriage?" was the way she summed it up.

The very fact that Benjamin and Trish had come in for therapy was good news. Despite the fact that they didn't have enough information about their predicament to get out of it without help, the willingness implied that they could imagine causes that were beyond their present ability to fathom.

The therapist's first inquiries of Trish were meant to discover any trauma in her relations with her primary caregivers when she was a child. Rather than trying to find out what her present experience of sexuality was with her husband or to find out what his part in her sexual retreat might be, it was important for the therapist to find out where in Trish's past her sexual attitudes had been formed. Had there been any experiences in her childhood that had been sexually traumatic for her?

Trish spoke about her most important caregivers, and soon she was able to identify a stepfather whose behavior toward her was crucial. Trish remembered being six years old. Her stepfather would open the door to the bathroom when she was bathing and "leer" at her. "Leer" was the word she used. She re-experienced the embarrassment, disgust, and fear she had felt. At first, she did not know how deeply she was affected. The therapist gave her the time to describe the way she was feeling, and eventually she gave in. She cried and covered her face with her hands. She could hardly breathe for all the sobbing. Benjamin was present as Trish expressed her childhood state and could feel how distressed she could still be made by this stirring up of her traumatic emotions. He was getting an introduction to the power of trauma to resurface in the present.

Trish was asked if the feelings she had toward her stepfather had an analogy with her feelings toward Benjamin when he was being sexual with her. She struggled against this painful truth but finally admitted it and owned it as a truth. It was a touching moment for all when Trish looked directly at Benjamin and told him this awkward truth. There was real power in that moment.

The triggering of this posttraumatic stress reaction by Benjamin's "leering" at her took her back to her childhood state, trapping her there and making her blind to the real emotions of her husband and incapable of accessing a mature response to them.

With the therapist's help, Trish recognized that when Benjamin approached her sexually, she was protecting herself from the emotional consequences of having been spied on by her stepfather; she went behind a wall, cutting off from Benjamin and justifying her fear behind a wall of contempt.

The therapist asked Trish if she had ever told her mother that her mother's new husband had been sexually abusing Trish through voyeurism. Trish said that she had not, because she hadn't wanted to cause her mother any trouble. Her mother and her stepfather were already fighting and she didn't want to make it worse, was the way she put it. In this way, Trish learned early on that speaking honestly about her sexual feelings was a threat to her security and might cost her the support of her mother and the family system to which her mother gave assent. She would suffer in silence. Retreat had given her dysfunctional safety and implanted its traumatizing template.

In therapy, with Benjamin's presence and support, Trish was encouraged to confront both her mother and her stepfather during chair work. She was encouraged to tell her mother why she had been frightened to tell her what was going on with the stepfather. Trish breathed deeply into the childhood feelings and released them, so that they did not stay bottled up in her as carried shame. She told her story clearly and for the first time. She told her visualized stepfather that his voyeurism was sexually abusive and how angry and worthless it had made her feel. She told him that she had been too frightened to tell him these things when she was six years old, but she was telling him now.

To her visualized mother she said that it was uncaring of her to always appear so overburdened that hearing her child's problems seemed likely to push her over the edge. She told her that her preoccupation with her husband made her an inappropriate mother. Trish said,

"I was so ashamed of myself because of how Stepfather looked at me, but I was frightened to tell you because you had your own problems. What problem is more important than your own husband sexually abusing your daughter? That is shameful, Mother. I know you did the best you could, but that wasn't good enough for me. You acted shamefully to me, and I took that shame on as my own and have carried it into my own marriage. It's time for this to stop. And I am stopping it right now. I give you back your shame. And I give back to Stepfather his shame. It was never mine."

Trish learned to direct her sexual problem toward the stepfather and mother who traumatically generated it, rather than at her husband. Because Benjamin had observed the work his wife was doing, he understood that what was going on with his wife's attitude toward sex was about trauma and not about her distaste for him or about her being a terminally irresponsive sexual woman. His need to defend himself against her was replaced by empathy. He was ready to cooperate in her recovery.

For his part, Benjamin was encouraged to share with Trish what it was like for *him* when she would shut down, but without blaming her for the sense of distance he felt. Here his talking boundary needed to be in place so that he did not fall into the blame-game trap. "When you retreat from me," he said, "I have these feelings." He described them without giving them any loaded emotional edge. He used his talking boundary. He did not blame.

One of the most important things for Trish and Benjamin in recovery was for Benjamin to speak up when he felt that Trish was reverting. He would say that it was his perception that she was falling away from him again, and he told her how he felt when that happened. He asked her to talk about what was going on with her.

She in turn started to share with him what was going on, but, rather than directing her attention at "what Benjamin *made* her feel," she shared with him the connection between her feelings and what she felt about her stepfather. She was learning to take full responsibility for her own emotions and not copping out by saying "Benjamin *made* me feel this way."

PHYSICAL TRAUMA

"It Wouldn't Kill You to Show Some Affection, or Would It?"

The couple complained of their difficulty when they wanted to express their affection physically. They were reluctant to touch or to stand close to one another and look deeply at one another. Marianne complained that Harvey never reached out to make contact with her, and she also noticed that whenever she reached out to touch him affectionately, like giving him a hug or rubbing his shoulders, he withdrew and acted as if what she was doing was making him uncomfortable or that she was being offensive.

Marianne said that they had two daughters and a son and that Harvey was rarely physically affectionate with them. The children would approach him and give him a hug, but he looked as if he didn't want to be touched, that somehow contact with his children was unnerving to him.

The therapist asked Harvey what his own experience was when his wife reached out to him for affection, and he admitted that he felt uncomfortable. After thinking about it more deeply, he identified his emotions as pain and fear.

The therapist encouraged Harvey to describe how physical affection was experienced in his family of origin. He reported that his parents hardly ever touched. He recalled that even when they were seated in the same room, they sat fairly far from one another. He could not recall their looking closely into one another's eyes. The only kind of physical contact that stuck out in his memory was when Harvey's father or mother disciplined him for having behaved badly.

Harvey was encouraged to share with his wife and the therapist what it was like emotionally for him not to have been nurtured physically by his mother or father. He reported that he felt very lonely and felt that there was something wrong with him. He recognized that as a child he had started to make up in his own mind that it was inappropriate to physically touch other people, because that was the message he was getting from his parents. Harvey saw how his discomfort with affectionate contact sent out signals to others not to touch him.

Marianne reported that in childhood her mother seemed to be normally physically affectionate. She gave hugs and kisses and picked her up and touched her hair when it was out of place. Marianne's father, too, had treated her with reassuring and appropriate physical affection, which, she remembered, made it all the more disquieting to her when he stopped almost all affectionate contact with her when she became a teenager. Not only did he seem consciously to avoid contact with her, but also he seemed very uncomfortable when she approached. She thought long and hard about this experience with her father, and the word she kept coming back to in order to describe this experience was that she had felt "abandoned" by him and that it had something to do with her becoming a sexual female. She reexperienced the pain when talking to the therapist and added that the experience made her feel worthless.

It had become clear that in the childhoods of each member of this marriage there had been trauma around the issue of physical affection. Each was encouraged to do chair work with his or her parents. Harvey shared with his visualized mother and father what it was like for him not to get any physical nurturing from them. He told them that he had made up that there was something wrong with him because they weren't physically affectionate with him. He imagined that he was defective. As he confronted them with the evidence of their physical abuse, he reexperienced the emotions he had had when he was a kid. He felt lonely and worthless. He was back at the place where his present feelings of worthlessness came from. For him today, when Marianne withholds affection he feels abandoned and defective. How does it come about that Harvey, who does not offer affection, feels abandoned when he does not get it in return?

Harvey's parents' neglect of him had covertly shamed him. Because their reluctance to touch him gave the message that there was something wrong with him, when he rejected his wife's advances, he was trying to avoid a shame attack. The presence of the affectionate act he had been missing dragged him back to the traumatic place where he had learned he was defective. He could neither give nor receive affection. In his chair work, he was encouraged to give his carried shame back to his parents.

Marianne did chair work with her father about how she felt when he stopped being physically affectionate with her when she became a teenager. She told him that she had felt pain and the worthlessness that came along with her feeling that he had abandoned her and that it had something to do with her becoming a sexual woman.

After her chair work, Marianne could see that some part of her reaction to her husband was connected to trauma instigated by her father. It is true, however, that some of her reaction to her husband had been born out of the considerable history they had accumulated of not being affectionate with one another and had, thereby, become self-fulfilling. To break the cycle they would have to "exercise" being affectionate through conscious boundary work.

The therapist encouraged the husband to start to approach the wife physically with affection and to share with her what emotions came up for him as he did this, relating these feelings more to what had happened between him and his parents than to the present experience of reaching out to her. Although he was very uncomfortable initially, he persisted in exercising his physical boundary as he approached her, and eventually his boundary practice gave him the experience of truth and respect.

As Harvey became more comfortable, the therapist had Marianne start approaching her husband for physical affection, with which initially Harvey was very uncomfortable. But Harvey could now recognize that a lot of his reaction stemmed from his childhood trauma. Because Marianne approached him with respect, he felt that he was in control of whether he got touched or not and would not be overwhelmed and thrown back into the place of trauma. Harvey started to move from a wall for a physical boundary, which cut off all intimacy, into a boundary that invited intimacy under the conditions of truth and respect. He became willing to be vulnerable.

Harvey started to practice approaching his children after he had gotten more comfortable approaching his wife. He did more physical nurturing with his physical containment boundary in place, reminding himself that the shame he felt when he was affectionate was a ghost of his traumatic past and could be breathed into and made to disappear. Through boundary practice, the conditions under which love and respect could grow were created and nurtured. There was no guarantee that practice would turn into enduring heartfelt intimacy, but there was hope.

INTELLECTUAL TRAUMA

Contempt: The Mask of Shame

Cal complains that he has lost respect for his wife, Donna. Cal says that Donna doesn't offer her opinions on anything: not when they have private conversations, not when they talk about politics or music or their friends, not even when they are out in public at a party. It annoys him that despite her withholding of any passionate opinion she seems liked by almost everybody. He accuses her of being a people pleaser, smiling into everyone's face at a dinner party. He admits how resentful this makes him feel—that her lack of intellectual conviction, which makes him feel distant from her, seems to make her universally thought of as "nice." He says, "What the hell is she frightened of?" Her insouciance often makes him feel like a boor by comparison. Emotionally and personally he feels that she has withdrawn from the relationship. He is feeling very lonely and depressed. He has been in AA for twelve years. He shares with the therapist that he may drink again.

In examining Donna's family-of-origin issues, the therapist finds strong evidence of a healthy intellectual environment. Her mother and father exchanged ideas freely, and she remembers enjoying their conversation and being welcome to offer her own opinions. Donna admits that she is not as intellectual as Cal, and it is her style to enable conversation, not initiate or dominate it. Without seeming to compliment her husband falsely, she says that she thinks he is a genius and sees very little reason to take up intellectual space that can be better occupied by him. She says these things confidently, with good self-esteem, and with becoming modesty. Nonetheless, she believes that Cal is in crisis and that he is assigning the blame to her. She fears for the relationship, which she treasures.

The therapist discovers that in Cal's childhood he was the object of his mother's smothering love. For her he was a god and her worth came from his reflected glory. He was the smartest, the most handsome, and the best. Cal's father, a workaholic and an isolator, was hardly ever at home, and when he was, the mother and father raged at one another obscenely, with the threat of violence always in the air. All the mother's affections were transferred to her only son, Cal. She made it known to Cal that her life depended on his love for her. She taught him in return that his safety was entirely wrapped up in her well-being.

On one hand, the son was being falsely empowered by his mother, made into a little god. However, it was clear to everyone who knew the mother that she was manic-depressive, could not think logically, and was so emotional that she was often a social embarrassment, spewing emotion in every direction. Having a sane conversation with her was often impossible. Emotion ruled her. Sometimes she would cry with joy because the sun was out. At other times she would cry at the sight of a traffic accident on the nightly news. Cal told the therapist that one weekend at their country house, when he was fed up with her brutal cooking, he had tried unsuccessfully to teach her to associate the temperature on a meat thermometer with the doneness of the chicken. One thing her mind was clear about was that her life depended on Cal and that Cal was a god. To this day, when meat is overcooked, Cal feels deep pain.

By the time Cal was twelve years old, he realized that his mother was a sick person and that therefore his sense of superiority came from a very suspect source. But the god role had been implanted before he was five years old. It was in his soma. Nothing short of godlike behavior would allow him to fulfill the role his mother had set him up to play, while simultaneously he felt that his empowerment was fraudulent. If he spoke like a god, it would be a lie. If he admitted that his authority was counterfeit, he would betray his mother and have a shame attack.

Running from the insanity of his unacceptable background and using his family's considerable wealth, he had become a university teacher noted for his genius and clarity of expression. He dressed like an English gentleman and drank like three of them. By the time he was thirty-eight, he had been in several detoxes. His third DWI had brought him into AA. He had been sober twelve years now. His marriage to Donna was in its twenty-fifth year. They had three children, all of whom were in good colleges. His mother had just died. He had been unable to mourn her loss.

In doing chair work, the image of Cal's mother in the room would make this cultured, elegant, well-spoken man sputter. He would scream at her that she understood nothing that he said. He told her that he could have been born without a brain and she would still have told him he was her baby Jesus. But her lack of a real husband didn't give her the right to take over his soul and use it to fulfill her own desperate need to be loved.

The therapist asked him what emotion he felt when his wife, Donna, didn't offer an opinion or refused to join him in the intellectual fray. He said "contempt." He was asked what in his wife's intellectual withdrawal he found contemptible. He said that she didn't have a true voice, that she would not offer up her true feelings. What was it like for him to not have his true thoughts and feelings understood? the therapist probed. Did he have to deal with those feelings when his mother was bringing him up?

"Every day of my life," Cal said. That was the way he had felt every time he opened his mouth.

At this point Cal spoke without any more prodding from the therapist, almost as if he had just found a script he had carelessly left in his jacket pocket and had forgotten for many years:

> "So when I see someone who seems to be intellectually lost or unresponsive, it reminds me of my own child-hood inability to communicate and to be heard. What I do is delude myself into believing that what I am feeling is contempt, because contempt makes me feel superior, and my mother made my feeling superior the require-ment of my being a god. But what I really am feeling is shame—shame that I am a god without a portfolio—someone who has not been prepared by his parents to

know anything. I'd rather hold you in contempt than experience my own voicelessness and shame at powers I do not have."

Donna watched this startling epiphany of self-knowledge and was stricken with empathy for the painful knots into which her husband had tied himself. Donna's self-esteem was good, and she knew that her husband's struggle was not the result of any abusive behavior on her part. But she had lived with him for twenty-five years and seen him almost die of alcohol abuse. She had given him respect and love, and yet he was still enthralled to his trauma. She was in pain and she was frightened.

Donna and Cal agreed that Cal was at a crisis in his recovery. The therapist recommended that Cal go for extended in-patient treatment, which he was willing to do. The insights of which he saw the first glimmerings in couples therapy were nurtured and took hold. Nowadays, at his therapist's suggestion, the word "contempt" is in his morning prayer.

EMOTIONAL TRAUMA

Rage: Noisy and Silent

Two men come in for counseling. Guy complains that his partner, Steve, rages at him. Guy feels superior to Steve, whose rage Guy finds juvenile; it always lowers Steve in Guy's eyes. Nonetheless Steve's rage frightens Guy.

For his part, Steve complains that Guy is often withdrawn and silent. Steve makes attempts at conversation, but Guy will not be drawn out. Pretty soon Steve finds himself yelling in order to provoke some response in Guy. Steve goes into a rage.

In Steve's family of origin the father was a rager. Steve remembers how he learned to rage just like his father.

Guy's father was also a rager, on account of which Guy disliked him and kept his distance. Guy leaned on his mother, who sympathized with Guy's being raged at by his father and shared with her son that she thought the father's behavior was terrible. Guy's only experience of anger when he was a child was when it came from his raging father or was being disapproved of by his sympathetic mother. Guy grew up believing that all anger was inappropriate and offensive.

In his relationship with Steve, Guy—who believed that to express anger at all was to be an offender—was incapable of expressing his anger through his talking boundary. Instead, he stuffed his anger and refused to express it, believing that if he didn't do so, he would be just as offensive and cruel as his father and thereby offensive to his mother also.

When Guy stuffed his anger, Steve exploded, imitating the boundaryless rage of his own father, whose rage Steve had imitated as a child. Since carried anger will be provoked as effectively through stuffing as it will through explosion, Guy's stuffing his anger set off Steve's rage just as effectively as if Guy had ranted at him. Guy had learned from his mother and his father that to express anger was abusive and inappropriate. Steve had learned from his father to have no boundaries with someone who expressed anger of any kind, whether through explosion or stuffing.

During chair work Steve did rage reduction work with his father, confronting him about raging inappropriately and how Steve was made to absorb the carried anger. Steve "gave back" to him his father's shameful behavior and its legacy of carried anger. Steve told his father that the anger and shame were his, not Steve's, and that Steve would carry them for him no longer.

Guy needed to learn the difference between abusive aggression and legitimate assertiveness. He learned to give himself permission to express his anger assertively through use of his talking boundary, which empowered him to be honest with Steve and, therefore, intimate.

Guy then confronted his mother about giving him the idea that to express anger was inappropriate because it resembled his father's behavior. For her to have treated her son as if he were more mature than her husband, the boy's father, was falsely empowering him to judge his father without giving Guy the tools to understand his father's behavior. Too immature to understand the difference between abusive aggression and assertive self-esteem, Guy became traumatized around the issue of anger and brought the issue of "stuffed" anger into his relationship with Steve.

Working with the two of them, the therapist sensitized Steve to those occasions when Guy was clamming up. Steve comprehended that he would become infected by Guy's stuffed anger and become primed for a rage attack. Steve, now aware of the psychodynamics of the anger issue, learned to breathe into the carried anger and to dissipate its poisons, freeing him to come out from behind his wall of anger.

Guy was encouraged to check himself all the time, noting when he was angry and expressing that directly to his partner through the talking boundary.

In a surprisingly short time the rage cycle was broken, and with appropriate boundaries in place Steve and Guy were able to enjoy the intimacy they had sought from one another.

10

PIA'S RELATIONSHIP MAXIMS

God is good, but our parents are screwed up. Given those two truths, we have our lives to look forward to.
—Anonymous

1. *You cannot "nice" someone into a relationship.*
When you are being nice to a person instead of being real, you are not in the truth of who you are. You are being manipulative, creating the illusion of a relationship disguised behind the "mask of nice." Since the mask of nice does not offer truth and intimacy, it is nonrelational.

2. *You can't be distant and caring. When you care for someone, you are there for that person.*
You have to show up and pay attention. You have to be responsive and stay involved. Care most often requires hands-on involvement. In this case, distance, rather than "making the heart grow fonder," makes the heart more distant. Are you one of those people who leaves the sick friend's hospital bed to watch the Academy Awards?

3. *If you are judgmental, your value system may be too big.*
If you've got a whole lot of things you think are right or wrong,

you are going to disapprove of a whole lot. When we notice people operating outside our value system, the first thing we do is to get judgmental. We make up that those people are bad people, and we go into the one-up position, looking down at those "wrong" people. We are left with a big value system and a small number of friends.

4. *Our own experience of shame makes it possible to be relational.*

When we experience our own shame, we believe that someone has seen us as we really are—human and imperfect. When you can feel your own shame, you know that you are not a god or a goddess. It keeps you from being judgmental toward your partner and helps you speak with humility. It keeps you the size you really are. Humility is recognizing both our weaknesses and our strengths. It is not about denying our values.

5. *We choose our behavior. The world chooses our consequences.*

We do not know what the consequences of our behavior will be, and we cannot control outcomes, only inputs. The consequences come as a result of whatever the people around us think about what we have done and how they act in turn. Chance also enters in, and we can control neither others nor chance. The expression "Let go and let God" has the truth of this maxim at its center, and so does the concept of "surrender."

6. *Date only the people you admire enough to criticize.*

Dating should be about finding out who our potential partner is. But when we date and find someone we really like, rather than putting in the time to find out who he or she really is, we spend our time ignoring that. We focus only on the parts of our date that we find pleasant and try to dismiss the rest. As the relationship ages, the opposite happens, and we focus on what we don't like and ignore what we do.

7. *Lead your life and see who shows up.*

Finding a partner shouldn't be about hunting. When you're leading your life in accordance with your authentic self, you are confident and relaxed enough to wait for the right person to show up. Health attracts health. Your calmness is a form of serenity and faith and makes you attractive. The people attracted to you will be so for all the right reasons.

8. *When walled-in people develop healthy boundaries, they will at first feel naked and vulnerable.*

When you are using walls for a boundaries, you have placed yourself in a state of invulnerability. Nothing can get to you. Nothing offends you, and you offend no one. The sense of power in invulnerability is a delusion maintained behind walls. It keeps you out of relationships and keeps you alone. When you have become used to this state of invulnerability, the disappearance of walls and the substitution of boundaries will make you feel naked by comparison.

9. *Resentment is like taking poison in the hope that your enemy will die.*

Resentment is victim anger. Self-pity is victim pain. Both are normal emotions, and they are not toxic if in fact we have been the object of a boundary violation. Resentment and self-pity are important when we feel someone has wronged us and treated us as if we were worthless. Resentment and self-pity help us go to a proper defense. But when we *falsely* feel that we are victims, when we feel the need to get even with someone who has *not* victimized us, we become obnoxious and self-defeating. If, for example, our partner has just made an erudite remark about the opera and we resent him or her for being "arrogant," that is just a failure of our own self-esteem. Just because something has gone badly for us—we didn't get invited to a party or our term paper didn't get a good grade or bad weather spoiled our vacation—does not mean our boundaries have been violated. To feel resentment and self-pity in the latter cases becomes a self-inflicted poison and makes us our own tormentor.

10. *Getting esteem from someone else never creates self-esteem.*

Self-esteem is generated from within. The esteem we receive from others is other-esteem, and it varies according to those from whom it is received. Self-esteem that stems from our awareness of our inalienable and unvarying worth is not subject to the vagaries of the judgment of others.

11. *Sex is not the equivalent of a handshake or emptying your bladder.*

Since it is easier to be sexual without vulnerability than with it, object sex can become a pernicious habit and infect lovemaking even with someone about whom you care deeply.

Using sex to introduce yourself to somebody is not good self-care, because you don't know the person well enough to be doing something that intimate. Becoming emotionally vulnerable with someone you don't know is dangerous. It is also spiritually cynical to use sex like a convenient discharge of effluents.

12. *Setting up a boundary with those who are boundaryless makes them feel abandoned.*

Boundaryless individuals are used to getting too close, used to being in another person's face, so that even the healthy moderate distance of a boundary threatens them. At the other extreme, when you ask persons who habitually use a wall for a boundary to let go of that wall and move into contained vulnerability, they feel too naked, too vulnerable.

13. *"When you resist my control, I feel abandoned."*

This is the way a lot of dysfunctional mothers feel about their children and one member of many dating couples feels about the other. "When I want you to be a certain way and you won't agree to do that, what I make up about that is that you don't love me, because if you did love me, you would do what I want you to do." A variation on this is, "When you use boundaries, I feel helpless." In other words, "When I try to manipulate you and you are using your boundary system, I can't and I feel helpless." This is a good reminder that properly boundaried people exert quiet but considerable force.

14. *Conditional love is immature love and never feels satisfactory to a child.*

The message of conditional love to a child is "I hold you in high regard only when you are busy being who I want you to be." The implication is "When you are busy being who you are, you are not lovable to me."

15. *A relationship with an unconscious person is impossible.*

This maxim is true in two senses. In one sense, no relational health will ever be achieved if one member is an active substance abuser. The other sense in which being unconscious precludes relationality is when dysfunctional people remain ignorant of their traumatic past and are, therefore, incapable of freeing themselves from its compulsions.

16. *A new relationship cannot begin until you have grieved the last relationship.*

Another way of saying this might be "Grieving only stops when it is over." If you get involved in a new relationship before the grief period for the old one has ended, the thoughts and emotions still left unresolved because of incomplete grieving will poke themselves into the new relationship where they are inappropriate. Also, when you start a new relationship before you have ended another, you are likely using the new relationship to get out of the original one, an exit strategy that is manipulative and therefore nonrelational.

17. *It's easier dealing with the drunk you know than the sober human being you don't.*

This might be subtitled "The Codependent's Lament": "I was capable of handling you when you were out of control, but now that you are getting a grip on things, there may not be any need for me. If I no longer have to be the caretaker, what is there for me to do?" When a relationship is based on the need to care for, ameliorate, and deny the actions of an alcoholic, the caretaker may lose touch, not only with the humanity of the drunkard but also with his or her own.

18. *Love is about knowing someone matters. That way you can't love them too much.*

Loving someone for the right reasons means that you are giving self in a boundaried and self-esteeming way. Your emotion is free of manipulation. Such intimacy always reaches out for what is real in your partner. Of such love, there can never be too much.

19. *"I don't need your help to have boundaries."*

"My boundaries protect both of us: me from your perception of me—no matter how hostile—and you from my anger." This is a neat summing up of the function of the listening boundary, which protects us from incoming information, and the talking boundary, which protects others from what comes out of us.

20. *If we don't esteem ourselves, we can't believe another can love or esteem us.*

If we believe we are worthless, nobody is going to be able to convince us that we are lovable and have inherent worth, because what another would tell us is in too great a conflict with the bad stuff we believe about ourselves.

21. *Nothing in a relationship is improved by marriage.*

Marriage tends to intensify problems. Marriage is about committing to a person and a relationship. It is not about improving things. The obverse wisdom is "Everything in a marriage is improved by a relationship."

22. *There is no such thing as an illegitimate child.*

The circumstances under which a child was conceived might be debatable but never the value of the child.

23. *Much of recovery is acceptance.*

"I rarely get my way entirely. However, I do get enough to be comfortable."

24. *Comfort is not the average between extremes.*

As Albert Einstein observed, if you put one hand on a burning stove and one hand in the freezer, on average you will be comfortable. We don't keep a canoe on an even keel by first hurling ourselves to one side of the canoe and then to the other. Einstein understood the physical mysteries of the universe; it is mete that he would understand the spiritual ones as well. Living at the extremes of all our core issues is how we destroy our ability to have healthy relationships. Learning how to move to the center of each creates the supreme psychological blessing: *being centered.*

11

FINDING THE CENTER

At the still point of the turning world. Neither flesh nor fleshless;
Neither from nor towards; at the still point, there the dance is,
But neither arrest nor movement. And do not call it fixity,
Where past and future are gathered. Neither movement from nor
   towards
Neither ascent nor decline. Except for the point, the still point
There would be no dance, and there is only the dance.
I can only say, there we have been: but I cannot say where.
And I cannot say, how long, for that is to place it in time.
T. S. Eliot, "Burnt Norton"

This concept of being at the center is key to our spiritual well-being. Although spiritual well-being is often associated with a state of mind, I have come to think of centeredness as having the force of a physical law of nature, like gravity or the conservation of energy. When we operate out of the center of our core issues through the practice of boundaries, our self-esteem is automatically restored. If I were to draw the wheel of human life, at its hub I would put *centeredness*, and the spokes that radiate out from it would be the attributes of our authentic humanity. When that wheel is put into motion by boundary practice, self-esteem is generated, and we are back at the place of authenticity, the place we reclaim as our spiritual home.

The two grand lies children hear from parents are that they are "better than" or "less than." The truth is that a child, as well as every other human on the planet, has inherent worth. It is not a quality that bears comparison. It is an absolute value, and we all have it. We differ from one another, but not in terms of inherent worth.

Dysfunctional, immature parents abuse children when they give them the message that they are "better than" or "less than." When the message is that they are "less than," this disempowering abuse shames them. If it is falsely empowering abuse, children become exalted above their parents. They exercise more power than the parents within the dysfunctional family system and literally take care of them.

But whether children are abused and disempowered ("less than") or abused and falsely empowered ("better than"), whether they become the Scapegoat or the Hero/Heroine, they will be painfully damaged. Neither persona is their authentic self. The Scapegoat is a bad god. The Hero/Heroine is a good god.

Shamed children feel less than human—defective—and this perceived defectiveness is a pernicious lie. They live in a spiritual distortion in which they believe that they are defective and that God would never love them. Their counterpart, falsely empowered children, know no other god but themselves. It will become a crippling burden.

That original parent-to-child wounding causes deep spiritual wounding. In each of the core areas of their authentic self, these children will become unbalanced: they will operate from "less than" or "better than" with walls for boundaries or with no boundaries. They will be too dependent or antidependent. They will be confident of their truth or not be able to tell truth from lies. They will be arrogant or self-loathing, rigid or out-of-control, exuberant or withdrawn, overly mature or overly childish. These children will be in a spiritual skew, unable to find balanced emotional centeredness.

Damage to every core issue results in extremes: "less than," "better than"; no boundaries, walls; "I am a good person," "I am a bad person"; "I want others to help me," "I don't want any help"; "I am rigid," "I am a spewer." Recovery lies at the center of these extremes.

If you have no boundaries to contain yourself, you are a spewer. You feel you can do anything you damn well please—like a god without accountability. If you have walls to contain yourself, you are rigid. You become shut down, one-up, judgmental, and controlling. You become an oppressive god: "Sit down, shut up. I know what you need to do." Boundary work teaches us to modify these extremes.

It is in relationship that we get triggered. Usually it is someone close to us who triggers in us the extremes of the core issues and brings up trauma issues.

One of the things I do in relational work is to get my patients to understand where their principal wounding is. To use myself as an example, I have an infant wound because my mother failed to care for me as an infant. I have a wound inflicted at age three, when I was raped by a gang of boys. I have a wound inflicted at age seven, when I remember very specifically coming to understand that my father hated me. And I have a wound inflicted at age twelve, when I began to believe that I was totally alone in the world, without any kind of backup; and I was totally enraged about that.

I have sensitized myself to recognize that when something triggers one of those wounds, I begin to feel emotions associated with one of those childhood states. I can identify the emotion attached to that infant wound; I know how it feels when I go to the three-year-old's wound, which comes up when I am being sexual. I know what it feels like to be in the seven-year-old's wound, which comes up when I am being relational with an important man who I believe is looking at me as if I am "less than." I go to that twelve-year-old's wound when someone who is close to me has wronged me. I know that about myself.

I try to teach people to be able to identify when they feel themselves going to an old wound and becoming, say, an infant or a seven-year-old, so that they can instantly know they have been propelled into the extremes of their core issues. If they identify the feelings as having first been experienced at five or younger, they are "less than," boundaryless, "bad," overly dependent, and uncontrollably spewing. If the feelings come from an older age, they go one-up, walled in, "better than," needless and wantless, and rigid.

Sometimes it is difficult to identify the core issue in which you are dysfunctionally operating, but immoderation in any of the core areas indicates the age at which the abuse was originally received. When the dysfunctional emotion is being informed by a younger wound, you will act like a spewer: in control of being out of control. When you are being informed by an older state, you will be out of control of being in control. You will try to control everyone, including yourself or, if you had disempowering abuse, you will find yourself manipulating through overdependence.

The way you get a grip on yourself is to watch yourself going into the rigid or spewing mode. If you have knowledge of your own wounding, you know about how old your feelings are and how they were stirred up. You can reassure that child that there is a functional adult on board now who can teach the child to use boundaries and be protected from pain.

So it is that whenever therapists are straightening out the lies of "better than" and "less than" and guiding patients back to centeredness and the place of inherent worth, they are involved in spiritual healing. In therapy, recovering individuals move from a lie into the truth, and that activates the spiritual principle that God is Truth. Also, they learn to love themselves, and that activates the spiritual principle that God is Love. Any work that confronts the "better than" or "less than" of abusive childhood—whether you are dealing with boundaries or the issues of self-esteem, reality, dependency, or moderation—confronts a lie and changes it to the truth.

In order for us to learn the truth, we have to get ourselves into the right position to receive it. We cannot be caught up and distracted in defending ourselves or in attacking. We have to learn what it means to be contained. Whenever we contain ourselves during intimate communication with our partner, we are in the act of loving that partner and in the act of loving the truth of who we ourselves are. Whenever we exercise our boundaries to protect the truth of who we are from someone who is approaching us intimately, we are in an act of self-esteem, at the same time that we are esteeming the truth of who the other person is. Both acts are acts of love: love of self and love of another.

Boundary work within the reality issue enables us to tell the truth about who we are. That activates the principle that God is Truth. Boundary work within the self-care issue automatically activates a sense of self-esteem in which we learn to accept the truth of our own neediness. That activates the principle that our needs will be met and that God is Love. When we have learned how to properly moderate ourselves, our containment boundary encourages us to protect the truth of self and trustingly honor the truth of other selves: automatically we activate those two principles (that God is Truth and that God is Love). So all core work is learning how to live in truth and in living in truth learning to love self and others. All trauma work around core issues is deeply spiritual work.

Being spiritual tunes us into the energy of our authentic self. Call it remembering. It's like tuning in that station on the radio. It puts you onto the right wavelength, you communicate with God's energy, and you find solace and guidance, peace, grace, and love.

If spirituality is the highest end of our becoming healthy, real intimacy with our partners is the path that leads there. As we have seen, the obstacles to intimacy are created early in our childhoods, when on account of immature parenting so many of us are traumatized into becoming allergic to our own humanity—what I have called our perfect imperfection. The adaptations we make to disguise our sense of inadequacy follow us surreptitiously into our adult lives and make it painful for us to have healthy relationships that lead to intimacy. But we can learn to recover this intimacy through an understanding of our trauma histories and the practice of boundaries. We have the tools to achieve the intimacy for which we have yearned. In this sense, as I have already said, we can be reborn.

The everyday evidence of this rebirth will be the life-giving intimacy we will attain in relationship with our partners. If there were no greater gift, this one would be immense enough. But there is a greater gift, and that is of a Higher Power, and I wish you its encounter.

APPENDIX

FEELING REDUCTION WORKSHOP

There hung a darkness, call it solitude
Or blank desertion. No familiar shapes
Remained, no pleasant images of trees,
Of sea or sky, no colours of green fields;
But huge and mighty forms, that do not love
Like living men, moved slowly through the mind
By day, and were a trouble to my dreams.

—William Wordsworth,
The Prelude, Book One

I may not hope from outward forms to win
The passion and the life, whose fountains are
Within.

—Samuel Taylor Coleridge,
"Dejection: An Ode"

You are as sick as your secrets.

—AA maxim

CHAIR WORK

Feeling Reduction Work, or, as we refer to it at the Meadows, "chair work," is at the center of the healing aspect of trauma work. Many times in the preceding chapters I have given brief descriptions of how people in need of confronting their childhood trauma engage in chair work, but this most dramatic and individualized therapeutic experience is so powerful I feel readers ought to see a fuller picture of it. So I have placed it at the end of this book, where it serves as a demonstration in action of the theories and practices we have been discussing in *The Intimacy Factor*. What follows has been culled from the Feeling Reduction Workshops I have conducted at the Meadows. It shows not only what the experience is like for our clients, but what our counselors must know before they can perform their healing work.

GETTING STARTED

A therapist or counselor structures the group, secures permission to touch the client, instructs group members to set their boundaries, and processes feedback after each client's process. Components specific to Feeling Reduction Work include positioning chairs for the major caregivers who have been identified as offenders, Inner Child(ren) Work, Integrating the Functional Adult, List Work, and Feeling Reduction.

ANTECEDENTS TO FEELING REDUCTION WORK

Intervention strategies that serve as prerequisites to Feeling Reduction Work include

Client education regarding child abuse and childhood trauma
Client education regarding the primary or core symptoms
    of codependence
Debriefing regarding child abuse and childhood trauma
Diagramming the presence and strength of the Inner
    Child(ren) and the Functional Adult
Inner Child(ren) Work
Integration of the Functional Adult

Debriefing is an important precursor to Feeling Reduction Work. In debriefing, clients disclose pertinent information regarding their childhood. Also, during debriefing clients share information that enables the therapist to identify energy they carry for their major caregivers.

Prior to Inner Child(ren) Work, clients are diagrammed to assess the presence and strength of the Wounded Child, Adapted Adult Wounded Child, and the Functional Adult. As a preliminary to Feeling Reduction Work, the Inner Child(ren) are extracted, as applicable, as a function of Preintegration Work, and the Functional Adult is integrated.

Also, prior to Feeling Reduction Work, the counselor reviews the History of Abuse forms to determine how the client felt as a child regarding each recorded abusive episode and how the client feels now as an adult as he or she reflects on each episode. The counselor focuses on shame words and key phrases that indicate that the client experienced feeling "worthless" and records them for use in Shame Reduction Work.

SEATING ARRANGEMENTS

Group work takes place in a room that is long enough to accommodate a chair arrangement in a horseshoe or U shape. Two chairs are placed in the curve of the horseshoe, and the remainder in two rows forming the straight sides. The client doing Feeling Reduction Work sits to the left of the counselor in the curve; the counselor is to the client's right. Other group members occupy the chairs in rows.

An exception to this seating arrangement is when a counselor is working with a client diagrammed as an "All Adapted Adult Wounded Child," one who is not cognizant of or is in denial of the wounded part of the self. In this case the counselor may, as a planned intervention strategy, sit on the client's left. This will provoke the experience of the Wounded Child.

CLIENT PREPARATION

The client is instructed to seat him- or herself comfortably in the chair, with feet on the floor and hands on the thighs, and is provided with an adequate supply of tissues.

A REVIEW OF THE PURPOSE
OF FEELING REDUCTION WORK

The counselor explains to the client that Feeling Reduction Work is a process through which he or she will give back carried feeling energy that is being held for a major caregiver with whom he or she, as a child, was enmeshed. Doing Feeling Reduction Work releases that energy. One outcome of Feeling Reduction Work is that the client stops overreacting to normal life experiences and underreacting to any current adult abuse. Also, the client is reminded that he or she is in charge of the process and can stop it at any time.

Feeling Reduction Work is an individualized process. There is no right or wrong way to do it.

PERMISSION TO TOUCH

The counselor secures permission to touch the client who is doing Feeling Reduction Work, reviewing what he or she means by "touching."

Clients are informed that they are to let the counselor know immediately if the touching interferes with their process, they can withdraw permission for touching at any time, and if they wish support by touching from the counselor at any time, they are to let the counselor know.

EXAMPLE:

> Counselor: May I touch you to show you where I will touch you to support you if you give me permission to? May I touch you on the back—here? I might also support you by touching the front of your knee—here. Let me know if you prefer that I not touch you. Also, let me know if you want me to support you by touching you.

When asking for permission to touch the client, the counselor asks directly and specifically, "Is it okay if I touch you?"

INNER CHILD(REN) WORK

Chair Position

If it is determined to have the client's Inner Child(ren) sit in a chair, the chair is positioned at the beginning of Inner Child(ren) Work. A group member is asked to place the chair in its initial position, touching the client's knees.

If the client wishes the chair farther than an arm's length from him or her, a group member moves the chair for the client. The client is asked to direct the positioning of the chair to a location with which he or she feels comfortable.

EXAMPLE:

> Counselor: Position the chair where you feel comfortable
> with it. Not too close. Not too far away. If,
> as you are talking with the child, you want
> the chair moved closer or farther away, let
> me know and we can move it for you.

Body Position

The client is directed to close the eyes and relax with breathing.

Thinking and Feeling Blocks

The counselor asks the client what he or she is thinking and feeling and proceeds to identify and process thinking and feeling blocks.

EXAMPLE:

> Counselor: What are you feeling?
>
> Client: Anxious.
>
> Counselor: Go up in your head and tell me what you are thinking that is causing that anxiousness.
>
> Client: I'm scared.
>
> Counselor: Might you be worrying about how well you are going to do and what you are going to find?
>
> Client: Yes.
>
> Counselor: Which one?
>
> Client: I am worrying about how well I will do.

The counselor addresses any concerns identified by the client.

EXAMPLE:

> Counselor: Let me assure you that there is no right way to do this. There is just what is going to happen and that is okay. Concentrate on being authentic. Don't make anything up. If you are not feeling or seeing anything, just say, "I am not seeing or feeling anything." Tell it as it is. If you do not remember, just say so. That is good enough.
>
> This is an experience to help you get in touch with yourself. You cannot fail at it. It is progressive. You enter the process where you are.

After addressing each concern, the client is directed to center or relax with breathing. Then the client is asked what feelings he or she is experiencing.

EXAMPLE:

> Counselor: Breathe back into yourself and as you are
>   turning back into yourself, tell me what
>   feelings you are experiencing.

It is important that thinking and feeling blocks are dissipated before continuing in the process. Often, having clients identify and talk about their feelings is enough to bring them under control.

Child Feelings

If while identifying thinking and feeling blocks the client presents as experiencing child feelings from abusive episodes, the counselor may wish to have the client address the child feelings. As an example, if the client is experiencing fear due to childhood events, the client is coached to verbally acknowledge the fear.

EXAMPLE:

> Counselor: I want you to say, "I am feeling some child
>   fear—the fear I used to have in the presence
>   of my father because he was so scary."

Intense Feelings

If at any point in Inner Child(ren) Work the client experiences heightened intensity of any feelings, the counselor encourages the client to verbally acknowledge those feelings. The client is also asked to inform the counselor any time he or she experiences child feelings. If the client is experiencing child pain, the client is encouraged to weep it out. If the client is experiencing fear, he or she needs to talk it out.

Extracting the Inner Child(ren)

The counselor works with the client in envisioning and identifying his or her Inner Child. If there is more than one Inner Child, one child is focused on at a time.

EXAMPLE:

> Counselor: I want you to get in contact with your mind's eye—that area across your forehead where you create your internal imagery when you close your eyes. What I want you to do is look down inside yourself and see if you can identify any energy that would represent your Adapted Adult Wounded Child. Do you see anything there?

If the client does not respond, the counselor continues to converse with the client.

EXAMPLE:

> Counselor: There are many places in your body in which the energy can be located. It could be in your chest, your head, your abdomen. Tell me what you see.

The client is encouraged to describe the Adapted Adult Wounded Child. If the client is still having difficulty imaging the Adapted Adult Wounded Child, coaching continues.

EXAMPLE:

> Counselor: We have talked before about your having an Adapted Adult Wounded Child who is powerful. When you get into that Adapted Adult Wounded Child, how old do you feel?
>
> Client: Six years old.
>
> Counselor: You feel six years old. What I want you to do is see if you can envision yourself as a six-year-old. Can you see it?
>
> Client: Yes.

Once the Adapted Adult Wounded Child has been identified, the counselor asks the client to describe the child, and a dialogue is begun between the client and the child.

EXAMPLE:

> Counselor: What is her name?
>
> Client: Sally.
>
> Counselor: I want you to talk to her. Say, "Sally, I need to talk to you."
>
> Client: Sally, would you turn and look at me?
>
> Counselor: What is she doing?
>
> Client: Looking out the window. Her back is turned to me.
>
> Counselor: How are you feeling as you look at her?

Client:	Sad.
Counselor:	Ask her if she will turn and face you.
Client:	Will you please stop looking out of the window and turn and look at me?
Counselor:	Did she turn and look at you?
Client:	Yes.
Counselor:	Tell her who you are. Say that you are her, grown up, and you have come to take her out of that household.
Client:	Sally, I am you grown up and I have come to take you out of that place.
Counselor:	What is she doing?
Client:	She doesn't trust me.
Counselor:	Ask what that is about that she doesn't trust you.
Client:	Why don't you trust me?
Counselor:	What did she say?
Client:	You never did anything to protect me.
Counselor:	How are you feeling when you hear her talk like that?
Client:	Sad.
Counselor:	Ask her if she would be willing to come away from the window and sit in this chair across from you.
Client:	Would you be willing to come and sit in this chair that is across from me?
Counselor:	What did she say?
Client:	She said, "Yes."

The counselor directs the client to explain to the child what is going on.

EXAMPLE:

> Counselor: I want you to explain to her that you are going
> to do some work with her mother. It is about
> what her mother did that was abusive to her.
> Ask her if she would be willing to stand behind
> your chair while you confront her mom.
>
> Client: Would you be willing to stand behind the
> chair while I talk to your mom?
>
> Counselor: What did she say?
>
> Client: She said, "Yes."
>
> Counselor: Did she get up and move to stand behind
> your chair?
>
> Client: Yes.

If there is more than one Inner Child, the other children are extracted.

EXAMPLE:

> Counselor: Now what I want you to do is see if you can
> envision yourself as a fifteen-year-old and tell
> me where she is.
>
> Client: She is outside.
>
> Counselor: What is her name?
>
> Client: Her name is Sally.
>
> Counselor: What I want you to do is get her attention
> and ask her if she would come into the room
> so you can talk to her.
>
> Client: Can you come into the room so I can talk
> to you?

Counselor: What did she say?

Client: She won't come in. She is angry.

Counselor: Ask her if she would share with you what she is angry about.

Client: Will you tell me why you are so angry? She said, "Because of all the things that went on in the family."

Counselor: I want you to tell her that you are going to confront her mother about some of the things she did to hurt her and you want her to stand behind your chair so she can observe the process.

Client: Would you be willing to stand behind the chair while I confront your mom about some of the abusive things she did to you? She doesn't think I will be able to protect her from Mom.

Counselor: Tell her that you won't let her get in the line of fire.

Client: I won't let you get in the line of fire. I want you to be safe. She has some doubts, but she will do it.

Extracting the Wounded Child(ren)

After extracting the Adapted Adult Wounded Child(ren), the Wounded Child(ren) are extracted using the same format as with the Adapted Adult Wounded Child(ren).

The counselor seeks to find out from the client where the energy of the wounded part of the self, that part of the self that is dependent, "less than," and vulnerable, is located. If the Inner Child is outside the client, the counselor asks about the child's position.

EXAMPLE:

> Counselor: Harry, do you have a sense of the Inner
>   Child?
> Client: Yes.
> Counselor: Where is the child?
> Client: In the woods where he is safe.
> Counselor: Is there some reason why you decided not
>   to put the child inside you?

If the child is not within the client, the client is directed to ask the child to come into the room.

> Counselor: What I want you to do is visualize that child
>   in the forest. See yourself in your mind's eye
>   walking into the forest and talking to him.
>   Say, "Harry, turn around and look at me. I
>   am doing work about issues I have with your
>   dad, and I would like you to come with me."
> Client: Harry, I would like for you to come with me.
> Counselor: What is Harry doing?
> Client: He does not want to come.
> Counselor: What is going on with Harry?
> Client: He is afraid of Dad.

If the client indicates that the Inner Child is afraid of the offender, the client is asked if he or she is willing to protect the child. It may be that the child is absent from the client because the client is unable to protect the child. Therefore, he or she needs to be in a safe place such as a room or a hidden place. If the client indicates that he or she is unable or unwilling to protect the child or does not want to be placed in that position, work is stopped. If the client is willing to protect the child, the process continues.

EXAMPLE:

Counselor: Are you willing to protect Harry?

Client: Yes.

Counselor: Would you let him know that? Say, "Harry, during this process I will be there to protect you and support you." Say to Harry, "I'm going to confront Dad about what he did to you. I want you to witness this and not be in the middle of it. So I want you to get up out of the chair and stand behind me."

INTEGRATING THE FUNCTIONAL ADULT

Next, the Functional Adult is integrated so that the client is working out of or is confronting the major caregivers with the strength of a Functional Adult.

Imaging the Functional Adult

The counselor assists the client in imaging him- or herself as a Functional Adult. The client is asked to see him- or herself as a person in recovery with right vision with reference to the five primary or core symptoms.

EXAMPLE 1:

> Counselor: This is you as you esteem the self or have self-esteem—as you have boundaries—as you are being diplomatic and being inter-dependent—as you are being moderate.

EXAMPLE 2:

> Counselor: Now I want to do some imagery work about envisioning a Functional Adult. Have you done that work before?
>
> Client: No.
>
> Counselor: Okay. What I want you to do is pay attention to your mind's eye in your right vision. Okay, now what I want you to do is envision yourself the way you want to look and be when your core symptoms are in resolution. Can you envision how you might look, how you might be standing, and what your demeanor might be? Do you have a sense of when you create an image of that? Envision yourself as accepting, not pretending, nonjudgmental, loving of the self and others, having good boundaries, being diplomatic and interdependent and mattering.
>
>   Do you have a vision of what that looks like for you? If you do not have a vision of it, you have a sense of energy that you can feel.

Sometimes a client may have difficulty envisioning him- or herself as a Functional Adult. This may occur when a client has not previously thought about what he or she would be like with the core symptoms of codependence in resolution. As an alternative, the client can attempt to see or feel energy that represents the Functional Adult. Later, the counselor can work with the client on developing an image of a Functional Adult.

EXAMPLE:

Counselor: It probably is difficult because you do not have the exact image of what you want. You may need to do some work on that. You can do what you can do right now. You are not going to fail. You may be having some difficulty. Put whatever sense of energy you can into your chest area and that is good enough. You do not have to worry about it. You are developing this consciousness for yourself. As you gain more understanding of this, you will form a reality of it that is more concrete than it is right now.

Inserting the Functional Adult

The counselor directs the client to draw the energy and vision of him- or herself into the right half of the torso.

EXAMPLE:

Counselor: I want you to draw that energy to you and put it in your right chest. Is it okay if I touch your shoulder and your back and your side?

Client: Yes.

Counselor: It is that area between your shoulder and
your waist. It is from this part of your body
down to your waist—down your back to all
the way down your front—from front to
back—from the top of your shoulder to
your waist.

I want you to see that energy. Give that
energy power and light. Now I want you to
see yourself drawing that energy inside your
body. Lean a little bit to your right hip as you
do that. Lean into that energy and use it
when you confront your mother.

This process enables the client to become an advocate for the
Inner Child(ren) out of his or her adult persona and to do for them
what they could not do for themselves in the past. It is a self-advocacy
process. It empowers clients and teaches them how to be there for
themselves.

CHAIRS FOR THE CAREGIVERS IDENTIFIED AS OFFENDERS

After Inner Child(ren) Work and Integration of the Functional
Adult, the chairs for the major caregivers who have been identified as
offenders the client will confront are positioned. The client is
coached in adjusting the chair in which each offender will sit when
the client images the major offenders into the room.

Before beginning the imagery work with the offender, the counselor reviews with the client the purpose of positioning the chair.

EXAMPLE 1:

Counselor: Sally, what you are doing is setting a boundary
with your mother. When you are doing chair
work, you are setting your external boundary
that will hold your mom back. What you
think about when you are doing this is "How
far back does Mom have to be so she is not in
my face and I can't talk, and how close does
she need to be so that I do not feel I have to
lean forward to talk to her?" Put her at a
distance with which you can sit up without
leaning back or leaning forward.

EXAMPLE 2:

Counselor: Before we begin the process, I am going to
ask a group member to position a chair
against your knees. Then I will ask the
person to pull the chair back and let you
establish your boundaries. I want you to set
a boundary in terms of where the chair is
going to be. Establish the distance you need
between yourself and your dad so that when
you see him sitting in the chair, he is not so
far back that you have a sense that he cannot
hear you and you want to lean forward, and
not so close that it is hard for you to talk to
him and you lean back in your chair.

> What you are doing is setting an external physical boundary with him. Take all the time you want in doing it.

EXAMPLE 3:

Counselor: Harry, what I want you to do is open your eyes and look at the chair in front of you. Paul will get up, stand behind the chair, and put it in front of your knees. I am going to tell Paul to start pulling the chair back very slowly. When you see him putting it into a position that is at the distance you want it, tell him to stop.

After the counselor has given this prefacing information regarding the chair, he or she directs a group member to move the chair up to the client's knees and very slowly start pulling it back. Then the counselor directs the client to establish the position in which he or she wants the chair.

EXAMPLE:

Counselor: Harry, what I want you to do is envision your father in the chair. It is too far if you want to lean forward. It is too close if you are going to lean back. Tell Paul where to stop the chair.

When the client identifies the position of the chair, the person moving the chair is asked to sit in it.

EXAMPLE 1:

> Counselor: Paul, sit in the chair so he can feel it with
> energy in it. Sometimes when you do that,
> you find that it is too close.

EXAMPLE 2:

> Counselor: Paul, sit in the chair so Harry can see what it
> is like, so he can see you as his dad. Is that
> okay?

The client is directed to envision the caregiver sitting in the chair.

EXAMPLE:

> Counselor: Harry, picture Paul being your father.

If the client begins to pull back or starts putting the elbows up, it is too close. The person positioning the chair is directed to continue adjusting the position until the client confirms a comfortable placement. The client is reassured that, if during the confrontation with the offender, the distance of the chair becomes uncomfortable, the chair can be moved.

EXAMPLE:

> Counselor: If while you are confronting Dad you feel
> that he is too close, let me know and we'll
> move the chair. Dad is sitting in back.

CENTERING THE CLIENT

Since the client has opened his or her eyes to position the chair(s) and is no longer centered, he or she is directed to close the eyes again and begin centering.

EXAMPLE:

> Counselor: I want you to close your eyes again and do
> some breathing to relax yourself.

REESTABLISHING CONSCIOUSNESS
OF THE INNER CHILD(REN)

If the Inner Child(ren) were placed within the client's external and internal boundaries, the client is asked to reenvision the child(ren).

EXAMPLE:

> Counselor: What I want you to do in your mind's eye is
> look behind you and see your two children
> back there. Can you see them?
> Client: Yes.

THINKING AND FEELING BLOCKS

The counselor attempts to determine the presence of thinking or feeling blocks. If any are present, the client is asked identify and talk about what he or she is thinking and feeling. As applicable, the counselor addresses thinking and feeling blocks.

EXAMPLE:

> Counselor: I want you to breathe into yourself and tell
> me if any emotions are going on with you
> that you would like to share.
>
> Client: I am feeling crazy.
>
> Counselor: It sounds like you have some fear about
> being seen by the group and having them see
> you being off the wall. It is difficult having
> people witness your vulnerability. That you
> are willing to allow that to happen and give
> yourself permission to be in the truth of who
> you are means that you are in a moment of
> loving yourself and allowing yourself to have
> a spiritual process. Breathe into yourself and
> tell me what you are feeling.

If the client begins to talk in a low voice, it may be that, as a moderation issue, he or she has too tight a grip on the self. The counselor may wish to coach the client to talk louder.

EXAMPLE:

> Counselor: Harry, your voice is so low I can't hear you.
> You are in the fifth primary or core symptom
> of moderation when you do that. I want you
> to be present. You're the son. This is your
> father. You are the adult child. You have the
> right to be an adult and to be powerful in
> this room and with your father.

The counselor continues asking the client to identify his or her thoughts and feelings until the client is "at neutral."

EXAMPLE:

> Counselor: What I want you to do is to breathe into
> yourself and tell me if any emotions are going
> on with you that you would like to share.
> Client: I am at neutral.
> Counselor: You are feeling at neutral. So, you are ready
> to go?

When the client is at neutral, they move on to the next phase of Feeling Reduction Work.

SETTING BOUNDARIES

There are two components in setting boundaries for the client who is doing Feeling Reduction Work. The first involves directing the client to set his or her boundaries. The second is to have the client place his or her child(ren) inside the boundaries if the client has done Preintegration Work.

EXAMPLE:

> Counselor: What I want you to do is set your boundaries.
> The first boundary I want you to envision is
> a bell-shaped jar or whatever object you care
> to envision for an external boundary. What
> I want you to do right now is bring that

boundary down and around you and your
children. They should be within that external
boundary. Will you do that? When you get it
done, nod your head so I know you've done
it. Okay?

Now what I want you to do is envision the
internal boundary. The internal boundary is
like a jacket you might wear. I want you to
place your children inside the jacket so that
they are protected inside your internal
boundary. I want you to envision that. When
you get it done, I want you to nod your head
so I know that. If you have trouble, let me
know and I will help you.

If the client has difficulty, the counselor continues encouraging
and coaching the client.

EXAMPLE:

Counselor: Make the internal boundary like a big jacket.
Let the children stand there, poking their
heads out of the top. Make it whatever size
they need. Expand it behind you so all of you
can be comfortable. Be sure you extend it
down in front of you—as far down as it
needs to go. Remember the internal
boundary goes up and down.

GROUP MEMBERS SET THEIR BOUNDARIES

Next, the counselor directs the group members to set their boundaries.

EXAMPLE:

> Counselor: I want to remind the group to set your own
> boundaries with Harry as he does this.
> Remind yourself that this is about Harry, not
> about you. You do not have to climb into
> Harry's process. You can be an observer. If
> Harry's process becomes intense and you
> feel like you are being drawn into it such that
> you start feeling tearful, emotional, or
> miserable, envision an energy field between
> you and Harry. Push against his reality. Say to
> yourself, "This is about Harry, not about me.
> I don't have to climb into his process."

IMAGING THE OFFENDER INTO THE ROOM

After enclosing the child(ren) in the client's internal and external boundaries and integrating the Functional Adult, the client is asked to image the offender into the room.

EXAMPLE:

> Counselor: What I want you to do is bring your mom
> into the room. It can be at any age, as a
> young woman, middle-aged woman, or old

woman. What I want you to do is bring an image in the room that you can easily visualize. Have your mom come into the room and sit down in this chair in front of you.

Next, the client is asked to describe the offender. This includes what he looks like, such as the color of his eyes and what he is wearing.

EXAMPLE 1:

Counselor:	I would like you to visualize your father. Then ask him to come into the room.
Client:	Dad, I would like you to come into the room.
Counselor:	Is he in the room?
Client:	Yes.
Counselor:	What I would like you to do is describe your dad.

EXAMPLE 2:

Counselor:	Image your father into the room and tell me what he looks like.
Client:	Dad, would you come into the room and sit with us?
Counselor:	Did he come into the room?
Client:	Yes.
Counselor:	What does he look like?

THE OFFENDER'S BEHAVIOR

After the client has described the offender, the client is asked to describe the offender's behavior. Describing the offender and his or her behavior gives reality to the process.

If the offender is acting appropriately, the counselor directs the client to discuss with the offender why he or she has been asked into the room.

EXAMPLE:

Counselor:	What is he doing?
Client:	He is quiet.
Counselor:	How does he look?
Client:	He is just sitting there.
Counselor:	Tell your father that you asked him into the room to tell him things you could not tell him before—that he was not there for you.
Client:	Today, Dad, I want to tell you how I feel about some things. I want you to listen. I've not talked about this before.
Counselor:	Because?
Client:	Because I didn't want to hurt you, and I was afraid to tell you.

If the offender's behavior is inappropriate, the client is instructed to confront the inappropriate behavior exhibited by the offender.

EXAMPLE:

> Counselor: Here are some things you can say to him:
> "You are the parent, I am the adult child."
> "You are the father. I am your son. I have the
> right to expect you to be here for me." "Be
> here for me." "Sit here and be quiet." "Stop
> acting like a child. Today, you are going to be
> here for me."

This allows the client to affirm the self. It also empowers the
client. The counselor continues asking the client to identify the offender's behavior.

EXAMPLE:

> Counselor: I would like you to describe your father's
> behavior.
> Client: He has his arms crossed.
> Counselor: What I would like you to do is ask him not
> to cross his arms.
> Client: Dad, will you uncross your arms?
> Counselor: What is he doing?
> Client: Shifting around in his chair.
> Counselor: Did he uncross his arms?
> Client: Yes.

If the offender does not respond or continues to behave inappropriately, the counselor urges the client to continue addressing the
inappropriate behavior.

EXAMPLE:

Counselor:	Is she sitting in the chair?
Client:	No. She is standing behind it.
Counselor:	It sounds like she might be looking defiant.
Client:	With both hands on her hips.
Counselor:	Tell her to stop that. Tell her to put her hands down to her side and come around the chair and sit down.
Client:	Put your hands down to your side and come and sit in this chair.
Counselor:	Did she do it?
Client:	No.
Counselor:	I want you to look at her and say, "You're the mother. I'm the adult child. Today, you are going to be here for me."
Client:	You're the mother. I'm the daughter. Today, you are going to be here for me.
Counselor:	What is she looking like right now?
Client:	Dumbfounded. She's saying, "How dare you talk to me like this? Who do you think you are?"
Counselor:	Look at your mother and say, "Stop defending yourself."
Client:	Stop defending yourself.
Counselor:	"I am not offending you."
Client:	I am not offending you.
Counselor:	"I am not wrong to have you do this."
Client:	I am not wrong to have you do this.
Counselor:	"What I am doing is insisting that you be my parent today and that is not wrong."

Client:	What I am doing is insisting that you be my parent today and that is not wrong.
Counselor:	What is she doing?
Client:	She is arguing with me and saying things like, "It's too bad we can't all be perfect like you."
Counselor:	Tell your mother, "I'm not going to get in an argument with you and explain myself."
Client:	I am not going to get into an argument with you.
Counselor:	"I want you to keep quiet so I can talk to you about how in the past you abused me."
Client:	Keep quiet and listen to me.
Counselor:	"Be here for me today."
Client:	Be here for me today.

EXAMPLE 2:

Counselor:	"You are the father. I am the adult son, and I have a right to have you be here and be sitting here respectfully for me."
Client:	You are the father. I am the adult son. I have a right to have you be here and be sitting here respectfully for me and be respectful of my process and assist me.
Counselor:	"And not sit there and look like you have to defend yourself from me like I am the offender and you are the victim."
Client:	And not sit there and look like you have to defend yourself from me like I am the offender and you are the victim.

Counselors are careful not to allow the client to put him- or herself in a vulnerable position such as asking the offender for support.

EXAMPLE:

Client:	I need your support.
Counselor:	Don't say that. Don't tell him that you need his support. That puts you in a vulnerable position with someone you have to confront about some serious issues. What I want you to say to your father is "I want you to be here for me today."
Client:	I want you to be here for me today.
Counselor:	What is he doing?
Client:	Smirking.
Counselor:	What does that smirk mean?
Client:	That I am being weird and this is stupid.
Counselor:	How do you feel about that?
Client:	He always does this when I try to point out something to him.
Counselor:	Since your father is being offensive, what I want you to do is say, "Wipe that smirk off your face. This is not funny. This is serious business. I brought you into the room today to confront you about some serious issues from my childhood and it is not funny."
Client:	Dad, get that smirk off your face.
Counselor:	"I want you to be here for this process. I want you to be my father. I want you to be present and to respect me."
Client:	This is not funny. I want you to be present and to respect me in this process.

Counselor: What is he doing?

Client: Sitting there.

Counselor: Did he take the smirk off his face?

Client: Yes.

After the client has confronted the offender, he or she is again asked to describe the offender's behavior, and it is addressed as applicable. If the offender is persistent in exhibiting or maintaining childish, defensive behavior, the client may be taken through the process without the offender's cooperation. However, the offender's behavior is periodically asked about.

EXAMPLE:

Counselor: We can see that your father is so immature
             that he cannot stop what he is doing. But
             you can proceed with your work. If he
             gets too far out of control, I want you to
             confront him. Do that as you need to.

The counselor observes the client during the process. If his or her demeanor abruptly changes, inquiries are made regarding the change. As an example, if the client suddenly becomes quiet, it may be because of what he or she is imaging in the offender's behavior. The counselor asks the client what is going on.

The counselor does not focus undue attention, however, on trying to make the offender act appropriately. If the offender is immature, they will not get mature behavior on the part of the offender no matter what the client does. The counselor may address the offender's immature behavior with the client.

EXAMPLE:

> Counselor: I want you to notice how out of control she is. You are not responsible for that. I want you to think about how difficult it was to have her as a mom. Set your boundaries and observe her immature behavior. We'll keep talking and she can keep doing that.

After the client has confronted the offender, the client is asked what he or she is feeling. As applicable, the counselor works with the client's feeling(s).

EXAMPLE:

> Counselor: Now, breathe into yourself and tell me if you are feeling any tension.
> Client: Anguish.
> Counselor: Where are you feeling the anguish?

The counselor continues processing feelings until the client is at neutral and ready to proceed to List Work.

LIST WORK

With the client's list of his significant childhood caretakers in view to assist in prompting, the counselor coaches the client through it.

EXAMPLE 1:

Counselor: Harry, I would like for you to talk to your
dad about the time you were driving the hay
truck and how you felt about that. Start off
by saying, "When I was five years old. . . . "

Client: Remember when I was driving the hay truck
and you were on top loading hay? I hit a rut
and the truck lurched and you almost fell off.
You went into a rage screaming and cussing
at me. You yelled and told me how stupid
I was.

EXAMPLE 2:

Counselor: I want you to talk to your dad about when
he had his friends at the house to play poker,
and they gave you beer to drink until you got
drunk and couldn't even stand up and walk,
and they made fun of you.

Client: You had your friends over to play poker.
They were really tough looking and scary
and talked loud and were rowdy. I had to
wait on you and get your beer, and when you
got tired of me being around, you kept giving
me beer to drink. I didn't even like it. I got
drunk and your friends made fun of me.

Counselor: "It was not good for a child to be around
that."

Client: It was not good for a child to be around that.
And you had no right to treat me like that.

Counselor:	Tell him that you are angry.
Client:	I am angry.
Counselor:	"You had no right to do that to me."
Client:	You had no right to do that to me.

EXAMPLE 3:

Counselor:	Go back and think of a time you tried to reach out to your mother.
Client:	I remember a time I tried desperately to reach out to you. I was four years old and came in after playing outside. I was hot and tired and had turned my tricycle over. I was really hurting and bruised and scratched up and wanted you to hug me, and you pushed me away.
Counselor:	Tell your mother that you were hurt and you wanted her to comfort you.
Client:	Mom, I was hurt and wanted you to comfort me.
Counselor:	"And you did not connect with me."
Client:	And you did not connect with me. I was the one reaching out for comfort.
Counselor:	How did that feel?
Client:	I felt confused. I felt empty and that I did not matter.

Statements such as "I did not matter" indicate that the client has "carried shame." The counselor addresses a client's shame by using the format for Shame Reduction Work. If it is the client's own feeling, the feeling itself is addressed. If it is fear, the client is urged to breathe it out.

EXAMPLE 1:

Counselor:	What are you feeling?
Client:	Fear.
Counselor:	What is causing that fear?
Client:	Just thinking about the situation. I fear what will happen.
Counselor:	That is that little-boy fear. That fear you had about not being able to see the ground and your father getting hurt because he was asking you to do the impossible. He set it up. It was not about you. You had a lot of fear as a child. Breathe in. Breathe that fear out. Can you see yourself doing that?

EXAMPLE 2:

Counselor:	Harry, I want you to confront your mother about your earliest memory of being in the swing. I want you to share with her what went on for you, how you felt then, and how you feel now. Go ahead and describe that in detail to your mom, starting off with, "Mother, I remember that time when I was two years old and you would swing me in the swing set." Tell her what happened to you.
Client:	I remember when you would take me out in the yard to play and would swing me on the swing and would swing me too high. I was scared and screamed, and you kept swinging me higher, and I fell out of the swing. I was terrified.

Counselor: Tell her, "I am feeling that terror within me
             now."
Client: I am feeling that terror now.
Counselor: "That old child fear."
Client: That old child fear.
Counselor: Describe to her what that feels like in your
             chest.
Client: My heart is beating so fast and so hard I feel
             it in my chest and pulsating in my neck.
Counselor: I want you to breathe down into it—take the
             air you breathe in, wash it through your
             lungs, and breathe that fear back out. Do
             that slowly or you will make yourself dizzy.
             Say to yourself, "I am releasing that old toxic
             fear."
Client: I am releasing that old toxic fear.

To reiterate, if the client has pain, the counselor has the client weep out the pain to release it. If the client is experiencing fear, he or she describes it and talks it out. When the intensity of the feeling dissipates, the client's process is continued. If the client has trouble being angry or expressing it, the counselor coaches the client in expressing anger.

EXAMPLE:

Counselor: Sally, tell your dad that you have the right to
             be angry.
Client: Dad, I have the right to be angry.
Counselor: Again and louder.
Client: Dad, I have the right to be angry.

The counselor continues coaching the client. The counselor says phrases like "Again and louder," "Louder," "Raise your voice," "Again," and "Do it again" at the voice level he or she wants the client to imitate.

EXAMPLE:

Counselor:	When you talked to your father about this, what did he say?
Client:	He said that it was his house and he could do anything he wanted to. If I didn't like it— tough.
Counselor:	"And today when I think about that . . . "
Client:	And today when I think about that . . .
Counselor:	"I feel . . . "
Client:	I feel angry.
Counselor:	Look at your father and say that again.
Client:	You just sneered and said that it was just tough and what did I think I was going to do about it.
Counselor:	Now, look at him and say, "That was an inappropriate comment to make to me."
Client:	That was an inappropriate comment to make to me.
Counselor:	Again and louder.
Client:	That was inappropriate. You did not even listen to me. You did not care. You were more interested in defending yourself.
Counselor:	"When I think about that, I feel angry."
Client:	When I think about that, I feel angry.
Counselor:	"And I feel angry that you defend yourself."

Client: And I am angry at you because you are
              defending yourself.

Sometimes the client may be overwhelmed by the presence of the offender. This may be compounded if this is the first time the client has confronted the offender. If this occurs, the counselor assists by supplying the language for the client. In this process, the counselor is reparenting the client and teaching the client how to be a Functional Adult.

When clients confront offenders, the counselor monitors the process to ensure that the confrontation is appropriate. It is inappropriate to allow clients to engage in behaviors such as screaming or uttering obscenities.

There are exceptions to not allowing clients to engage in immoderate behavior, however. These exceptions depend on the severity and type of the abuse. Also, sometimes clients need encouragement to yell in order to establish a sense of righteous anger.

FEELING REDUCTION WORK

Feeling Reduction Work involves dissipating a carried feeling by "giving it back" to the offender. This includes

Coaching the client in clarifying the client's own feelings
Establishing the difference between the client's own feelings
    and carried feelings
Confronting the offender
Giving the offender back his or her feelings

SHAME REDUCTION

Shame Reduction Work is a component of Feeling Reduction Work. There are five phases in Shame Reduction Work. Phase 1 involves identifying carried shame. Phases 2, 3, and 4 involve the client's verbalizing a set of phrases designed to eradicate the energy of the carried shame. Phase 5 involves the client's visualizing and transmitting the carried shame to the offender.

Phase 1

Phase 1 is composed of identifying carried shame and clarifying client's feelings regarding the abusive episodes and the offenders.

In evaluating the presence of carried shame, the counselor refers to shame words and phrases recorded in the client's List Work, adapting the feeling statements to the client's situation and prompting the client if he or she is having difficulty remembering the phrases.

A client's statement that he or she does not and/or did not matter is an indicator that the client has carried shame.

EXAMPLE:

Client: And you did not connect with me. I was the
            one reaching out to you for comfort.
Counselor: How did that feel?
Client: I felt confused. I felt like I just did not matter.
Counselor: Harry, when that happened did you feel
            worthless? Did you feel shame?
Client: Yes. I felt like I couldn't do anything right.

Phase 2

In Phase 2 the client verbalizes phrases that further acknowledge the shame and begins to give the shame back to the offender. The phrases used in this phase consist of the following:

> "You shamed me."
> "And your shame made me feel [the client's words reported regarding the episode]."
> "About that I am angry."
> "I have a right to be angry."
> "And I give you back your shame."
> "I will not feel [the client's words reported regarding the episode and in the first statement] for you any longer."

The client is directed to repeat the sentences one at a time through the counselor's prompting.

EXAMPLE 1:

> "You shamed me."
> "And your shame made me feel as if I did not matter."
> "About that I am angry."
> "I have a right to be angry."
> "And I give you back your shame."
> "I will not feel that I don't matter for you any longer."

EXAMPLE 2:

> "You shamed me."
> "And your shame made me feel as though I couldn't do anything."

"About that I am angry."
"I have a right to be angry."
"And I give you back your shame."
"I will not feel like I cannot do anything for you any longer."

The counselor coaches the client through the Phase 2 statemento.

EXAMPLE 1:

Counselor:	Look at your father and say, "When you did that, you shamed me."
Client:	Dad, when you did that, you shamed me.
Counselor:	"And your shame made me feel as though I couldn't do anything."
Client:	And your shame made me feel as though I couldn't do anything.
Counselor:	"About that I am angry."
Client:	About that I am angry.
Counselor:	"I have a right to be angry."
Client:	I have a right to be angry.
Counselor:	"I give you back your shame."
Client:	I give you back your shame.
Counselor:	"I will not feel inadequate for you any longer."
Client:	I will not feel inadequate for you any longer.

EXAMPLE 2:

Counselor:	Look at him and say, "You did not support me through that difficult experience."

Client: You did not support me through that difficult
               experience.
Counselor: "And your lack of support shamed me."
Client: And your lack of support shamed me.
Counselor: "And your shame made me feel dumb and
               bad and inadequate."
Client: And your shame made me feel dumb and bad
               and inadequate and stupid and a failure, and
               that I was never good enough.
Counselor: Tell him, "About that I am angry."
Client: About that I am angry.
Counselor: "I have a right to be angry."
Client: I have a right to be angry.
Counselor: "And I give you back your shame."
Client: And I give you back your shame.
Counselor: "I will not feel bad and inadequate and stupid
               and not good enough for you any longer."
Client: I will not feel bad and inadequate and stupid
               and not good enough for you any longer.
Counselor: Okay, now look at him and say, "You shamed
               me when you did that."
Client: You shamed me when you did that.
Counselor: "And your shame made me feel. . . . "
Client: And your shame made me feel bad and
               inadequate and dumb and stupid and a failure
               and just not ever good enough.

The counselor continues coaching the client until the client can do it without support. Minimal encouraging phrases like "Do it again," "Again," "Let it come up again," and "Again. The whole thing" are used to have the client repeat the shame litany. When the client has mastered repeating the sentences, the client is encouraged to go on without coaching.

EXAMPLE:

> Counselor: Harry, tell your mother, "You shamed me," and take it over. If you get stuck, I will supply the words for you. Go on your own.

Phase 3

When the client gets the rhythm of the phrases from Phase 2, the phrases are shortened to the following:

"You shamed me."
"About that I am angry.
"I have a right to be angry.
"And I give you back your shame."

The counselor continues verbalizing the phrases and coaching the client in repeating the phrases.

EXAMPLE:

Counselor: I want to hear you say, "You shamed me."
Client: You shamed me.
Counselor: "About that I am angry."
Client: About that I am angry.
Counselor: "I have a right to be angry."
Client: I have a right to be angry.
Counselor: "I give you back your shame."

Client: I give you back your shame.

Counselor: Start at the top. Say to your father, "You
              shamed me. About that I am angry. I have a
              right to be angry. And I give you back your
              shame."

Carried shame energy from the caregiver creates inadequacy in a
client. That carried energy is reflective of the caregiver's inadequacy.
Therefore, the client is directed to repeat this phrase several times.

Phase 4

When the client becomes proficient at repeating the phrases in Phase
3, shorten them to these statements:

"You shamed me."
"I have a right to be angry."
"I give you back your shame."

EXAMPLE 1:

Counselor: Now, shorten it to, "You shamed me. I have
              a right to be angry. And I give you back your
              shame."

EXAMPLE 2:

Counselor: I want you to say to your mother, "You
              shamed me. I have a right to be angry. And I
              give you back your shame." Again, say all
              three things.

EXAMPLE 3:

> Counselor: Okay. Now, Harry, what I want you to tell
>   her is "You shamed me. I have the right to be
>   angry. And I give you back your shame."

The counselor uses minimal encouraging words and phrases like "Good," "Keep saying it," and "Again" to coach the client in continuing the litany until the client feels that he or she has gotten rid of the energy.

EXAMPLE:

> Counselor: Now, say that until you feel you have gotten
>   rid of that old slimy, worthless, powerless
>   energy. Say, "You shamed me. I have a
>   right to be angry and I give you back
>   your shame."

Phase 5

The purpose of Shame Reduction Work is to move the shame-bound energy. When the client has the litany down, the counselor directs the client to concentrate on the shaming energy that he or she carried in his or her body for the caregiver.

EXAMPLE:

> Counselor: Sally, while you are saying, "You shamed me,
>   I have the right to be angry, and I give you
>   back your shame," I want you to move that
>   shame energy up out of your chest, up out

of your mouth, through the external
boundary, and onto your mother's lap.

As the client develops the ability to release his or her feelings, the release of the carried shame is augmented by having the client visualize the shame. The client gives color and substance to the shame energy and then visualizes releasing it from inside the body.

EXAMPLE:

> Counselor: You have the yucky shame energy in your
> chest. I want you to see that there. I want
> you to look at your mom and understand
> that part of that is her shame. I want you to
> repeat, "You shamed me, I have the right to
> be angry, and I give you back your shame,"
> until part of the energy moves from her
> to you.
>
> Repeat that as often as you need to. You
> may say it five times. You may say it a hun-
> dred times in the next ten minutes. I am
> going to get out of the picture and have you
> say it and concentrate on that shame energy
> in your chest and your mother and what
> part of that energy is her carried shame and
> move the energy.
>
> Start with "You shamed me. I have the
> right to be angry. And I give you back your
> shame."

Single words or short phrases are used to encourage and coach the client. Since righteous anger moves shame, the counselor coaches the client to raise his or her voice to the level that accompanies righteous anger. If pain comes up or if a client needs support during shame reduction, the counselor acknowledges the pain and supports the client through touching.

EXAMPLE:

Counselor: It looks like pain is coming up. Let your pain come up and release it. I am going to touch you between your shoulder blades. Is it okay to do that?

Let yourself have your pain. She hurt you with all that. It looks like that pain is still coming up. Let it come up and release it. When it recedes, I want you to sit up and look at your mother again and say, "I am very angry that you did that to me. I am angry. I have a right to be angry. And I give you back the shame of what you did to me!"

Sometimes a client may try to control the upsurge of pain by modulating his or her voice. A client's voice may be weak or may not be projected. If this occurs, it is important for the counselor to work with the client on increasing the voice volume. Through creating intensity, the client will be able to release the child pain.

REDUCTION OF OTHER CARRIED FEELINGS

The reduction of other carried feelings follows the Shame Reduction format. If the counselor suspects carried anger, he or she asks the client how the offender handled anger and what the offender was angry about.

EXAMPLE:

> Counselor: Was your mom angry?
> Client: Well, she never showed her anger.
> Counselor: Do you think she was angry?
> Client: I always thought she was mad at Dad for
>   running around with other women. I would
>   feel it for her. I'd be so mad at Dad for what
>   he was doing to Mom.

This is an example of a child taking on the feelings for the parent.

When a client has carried anger, the client is coached in repeating the following phrase or similar phrases to move the energy: "Right now I am feeling anger. But part of it is yours. I will not carry it for you any longer and feel your anger. I give back your part of this anger."

EXAMPLE 1:

> Client: Mom, I carry your anger, your anger from
>   then. I give you back your anger right now.
>   Right now I am feeling anger. Part of it is
>   yours. I will not carry it for you any longer
>   and feel rage-filled or continue to feel like I
>   have toward men. I give you back your part
>   of this anger.

EXAMPLE 2:

Client: When you beat me, you beat your anger at women in me. I carry that anger. It makes me rage. I am angry about that. I give you back your anger. I have a right to be angry. I give you back your rage for women. I will not rage at women for you any longer.

The counselor coaches the client with the appropriate phrases.

Counselor: Say to Dad, "Right now I am feeling fear. Part of it is yours. I will not carry it for you any longer and feel afraid that I am going to hurt or kill you. I give you back that part of the fear."

Client: Dad, right now I am feeling fear. Part of it is yours. I will not carry it for you any longer. I will not carry it for you any longer and feel betrayed.

Counselor: I want you to look at your dad and say, "Right now I am feeling fear."

Client: Right now I am feeling fear.

Counselor: "Part of it is yours."

Client: Part of it is yours.

Counselor: "I will not carry it for you and feel your fear any longer."

Client: I will not carry it for you any longer and feel your fear.

Counselor: "I give you back your part of the fear."

Client: I give you back your part of the fear.

Counselor: "Right now I am feeling fear."

Client: Right now I am feeling fear.

Counselor: "Part of it is yours."

Client: Part of it is yours.

Counselor: "I will not carry it for you any longer and feel your fear."

Client: I will not carry it for you any longer and feel your fear.

The counselor assists the client in continuously restating the last statement until the client can feel the energy shift.

EXAMPLE:

Counselor: "I give you back . . . "

Client: I give you back your part of the fear.

Counselor: Again.

Client: I give you back your part of the fear.

Counselor: Again and louder.

Client: I give you back your part of the fear.

Counselor: Again.

Client: I give you back your part of the fear.

If a client is having problems projecting, the counselor coaches the client.

EXAMPLE:

Counselor: Lean forward and really look at your father. Energize your voice a little more. I want you to physically lean forward. Look at your dad like you are an empowered person. When I think about a five-year-old trying to drive a hay truck in a rough, bumpy field, I am appalled. I can't imagine a five-year-old driving an old truck, especially with u man standing on top of a stack of bales. Screaming at a child for trying to do the task and for failing is ridiculous. You have a right to be angry about that. Look at your father and say, "Dad, you tried to make me do the impossible."

Client: Dad, you tried to make me do the impossible.

Counselor: "About that I am angry."

Client: About that I am angry.

Counselor: Keep repeating that.

The counselor continues to coach the client. After several repetitions the client is asked to describe what the caregiver is doing and then how he or she is feeling.

EXAMPLE:

Counselor: What is he doing?

Client: Sitting back in the chair.

Counselor: How are you feeling?

The counselor pays close attention to the client. If there are any changes in his or her behavior, those changes are checked out. If the client becomes quiet, the counselor asks what is going on.

EXAMPLE:

> Counselor: Tell me what is happening with your dad
> right now.
>
> Client: He is surprised and cannot believe that I am
> doing this.

If the caregiver's behavior is inappropriate, the behavior is confronted.

EXAMPLE 1:

> Counselor: Tell me what is happening with your dad
> right now.
>
> Client: He is looking at me strangely as if I am doing
> something wrong.
>
> Counselor: Say, "Dad, stop it. You're the parent. I'm the
> daughter. Today you are going to be here and
> not make it wrong and not make it about me
> that you would not connect."

EXAMPLE 2:

> Counselor: Tell your father that he is here today as your
> father. You are his daughter. Tell him his
> behavior is inappropriate and that you are
> no longer going to allow him to deny your
> reality or your feelings. He is here to sit and
> listen to you and not to be inappropriate or
> blame you, make you wrong or make you
> feel worthless.

EXAMPLE 3:

> Counselor: Tell him that what you want him to do is to
> sit there and listen and that this is your time
> to be able to tell him all that you have been
> unable to tell him and he is not to blame
> you.

CLOSING

When the counselor and client have completed the List Work or the time is up, the client is informed that his or her process is going to stop. The counselor directs the client to ask the offender to leave the room.

EXAMPLE 1:

> Counselor: Harry, would you tell your father that you
> are finished talking to him and ask him to
> please leave the room?
> Client: Dad, would you leave the room?

EXAMPLE 2:

> Counselor: Is there anything more to say to your
> mother?
> Client: No.
> Counselor: Then ask her to leave the room.
> Client: Mom, please leave the room.

When the client has acknowledged that the offender has left the room, a group member is asked to remove the chair in which the offender was sitting.

INTEGRATION WORK

If the relationship between the client and his or her Inner Children is functional, the Inner Children are integrated into the client and relocated into the area around the heart.

The client communicates with the Inner Children. With their permission, the children are asked sit on the client's lap. Then they are shrunken so they can comfortably fit in the client's hand. The client integrates the children into the area around his or her heart.

If there is more than one child, the client is asked which one he or she would like to work with first.

EXAMPLE:

> Counselor: Sally, what we are going to do now is integrate your child. Please explain that to your child.
>
> Client: I am going to put you in my heart where you will be safe.
>
> Counselor: Will you allow her to sit on your lap?
>
> Client: Yes.
>
> Counselor: Tell her what you are going to do. That you are going to make her very small and hold her in your right hand. Have her become small enough so if you clasped your fingers

	over her, you would not squash her—that
	small. Let me know when she is very small.
Client:	She is now.
Counselor:	Hold her over the left part of your chest.
	Have her enter your heart right now.

REORIENTING THE CLIENT TO THE ROOM

The client is then asked to concentrate on the breathing and, when ready, to open the eyes.

EXAMPLE:

Counselor:	Concentrate on your breathing and when
	you are feeling centered, slowly open your
	eyes.

IDENTIFYING AND ADDRESSING SHAME ATTACKS

If the client is experiencing a shame attack, he or she will exhibit behaviors such as slumped posture and covering the mouth. The shame attack must be addressed before working with the group, because a client will be unable to set boundaries with the group until the shame attack has been extinguished.

To address the shame attack, the shame bind that was a catalyst for the shame attack has to be identified. Then the counselor directs the client to look at a specific group member and verbalize his or her right to that behavior, thought, or feeling.

As an example, if the client has a shame-reality bind after expressing anger, the client is coached in verbalizing his or her right to express that anger.

EXAMPLE 1:

> Counselor: Look at Harry and say, "I have the right to express my feelings and be loud about it."

EXAMPLE 2:

> Counselor: Harry, look at Sally and say, "I want you to know that I have a right to be angry and I have a right to tell my father how I feel."

EXAMPLE 3:

> Counselor: Paul, look at Harry and say, "I have a right to be angry. I have a right to express that anger and I have a right to tell my mom that I am angry with her."

When the client can make eye contact, the shame has diminished significantly enough for the client to set boundaries with the group.

SETTING BOUNDARIES WITH THE GROUP

Before fielding feedback, the counselor has the client set boundaries with the group.

EXAMPLE:

Counselor: Harry, what you are going to do now is set
your boundaries in place so that you can
push away from anything that does not apply
to you and allow in whatever does.

FEEDBACK

In asking for feedback, the counselor tells the group members that
the feedback is to be their reaction to the process. If during feedback,
a group member experiences pain, the counselor addresses the pain.

If a group member begins to cry, the process is stopped and he
or she is given the time to do it. If a group member tries to resist the
pain, he or she is instructed to put feet firmly on the floor and the
counselor addresses feedback as appropriate.

INDEX